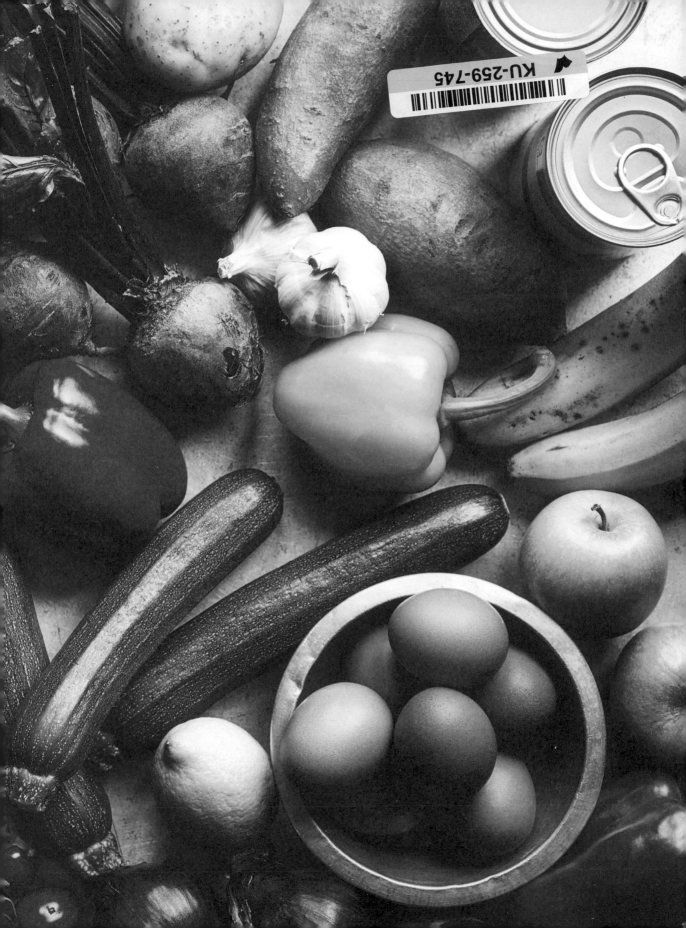

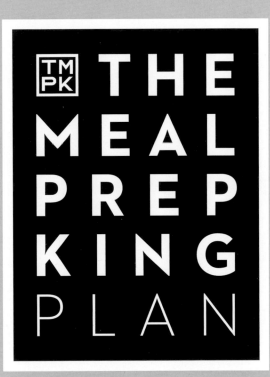

TM PK

THE
MEAL
PREP
KING
PLAN

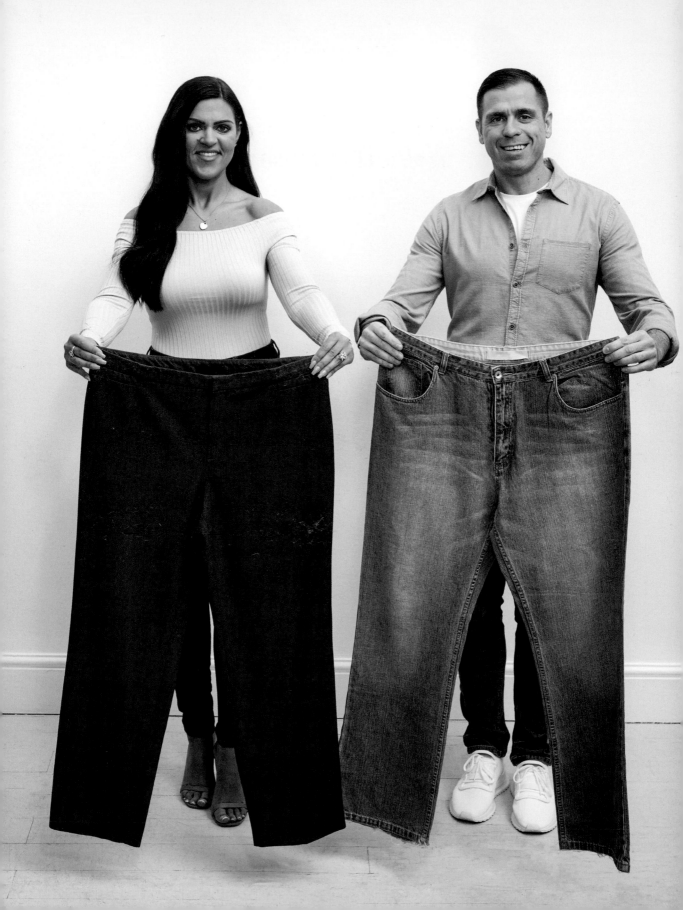

JOHN CLARK

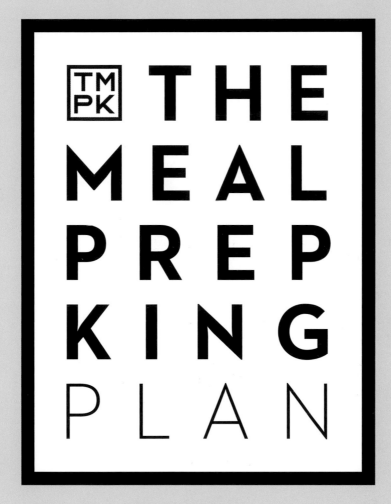

THE MEAL PREP KING PLAN

Save time
Lose weight
Eat the meals you love

MICHAEL JOSEPH
an imprint of
PENGUIN BOOKS

I would like to dedicate this book to Frank Barrow, the most important and influential person in my life.

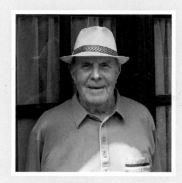

CONTENTS

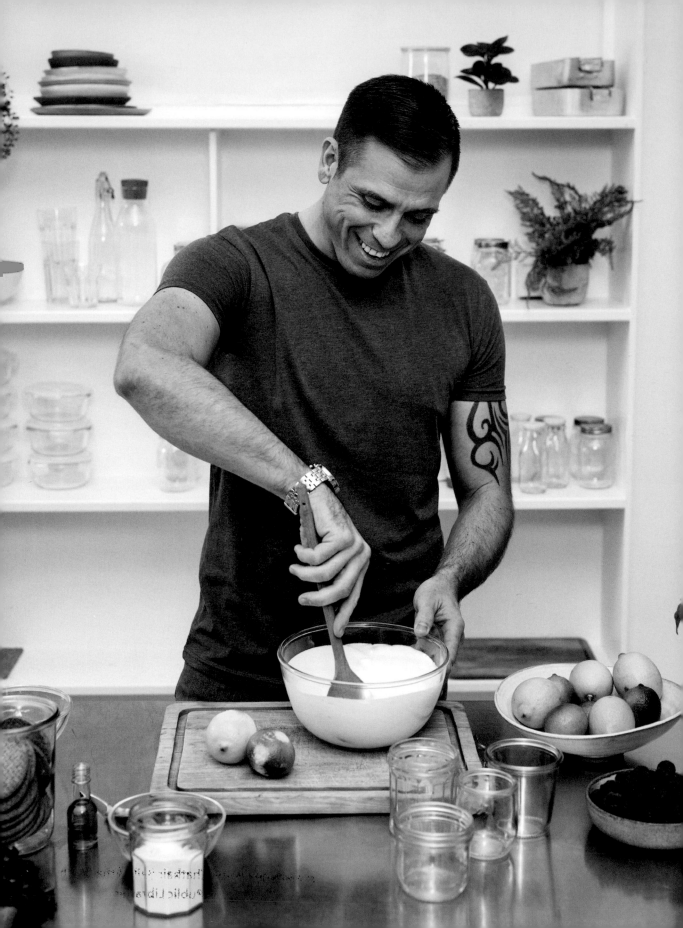

Hi there,

My name is John and I've been meal prepping for 18 years. In that time I've lost 9 stone in total and have discovered how to achieve permanent weight loss in an easy, healthy and affordable way – all because of meal prep. I've learnt how to 'prep my way back to health' whilst also saving money, time and food. Whether you want to completely overhaul your life or simply lose a couple of pounds, I'm here to show you how you can do it too!

I'm a 40-year-old based in Bolton, and my partner, Charlotte, who is 34, lives in Blackpool. Together we've turned our lifestyles around and now we are helping others across the world do the same. I've been cooking since around the age of six, often helping my grandad in the kitchen when I was a youngster. I've always enjoyed food and the endless possibilities that are at your fingertips with it. After all, one thing every human has in common is that we all have to eat!

Growing up, I wasn't an overweight child. In fact, I was a normal weight until I was about 21 years old, when I developed some pretty unhealthy habits including drinking too much alcohol and eating whatever I liked. My weight ballooned from 12st to 21st 6lb over the course of a few years. Often people told me I carried it well and looking back, I think this was the worst thing anyone could have said to me, as it gave me an excuse to gain even more weight.

It was a recipe for disaster and was starting to have an effect on my confidence, as well as many other aspects of my life. For one, my clothes were getting tighter and tighter. The usual high-street shops didn't really sell many clothes for plus-size people so I'd dread shopping trips. Everything I wore was black in an attempt to conceal how large I was. I'd end up taking 10 to 12 items of clothing into the changing room in a desperate attempt to find something that would fit. I was often stopped by security and told that I couldn't take in that many items at one time. I felt too embarrassed to explain why I had so many garments and, more often than not, I'd leave empty-handed. I'm quite a self-conscious person who likes to dress nicely and be well groomed, so not being able to find clothes that fitted was a big wake-up call for me.

I began to feel ashamed that I'd let myself get to this point, and when I hit my heaviest weight – over 21 stone – I realized that I had to do something about it.

I'd learnt about batch cooking from an old friend so I already knew how to avoid food waste and use everything up in my fridge. I started going to the library to find books about calories and the science behind weight loss. Armed with my new-found knowledge, plus a set of kitchen scales, a pen and some paper, I started to plan my food intake more carefully and soon I was shedding pounds of fat. I taught myself how to meal prep and cook in a way that meant I stuck to the necessary calories I needed every day and lost weight in a healthy, affordable and sustainable way, whilst also ensuring I didn't waste any food (I really hate food waste!).

Since then, I've sustained my 9-stone weight loss, grown in confidence and fallen in love with food for the second time – but in a much healthier way. I also fell in love with Charlotte along the way! Because of my weight-loss success, and having seen how much meal prep helped Charlotte too, I decided to set up an Instagram account to help teach other people how to make their weekly meals and show them that they too can transform their lives. A whole meal prep community has built up on Instagram and I absolutely love seeing people's creations and transformations. Now I simply couldn't imagine my life without meal prep.

In this book you'll learn more about me and Charlotte, our meal prep journey and how you too can change your life for the better with our tips and recipes to create a plan that lasts for life. Let's get started!

Thank you for reading,
John

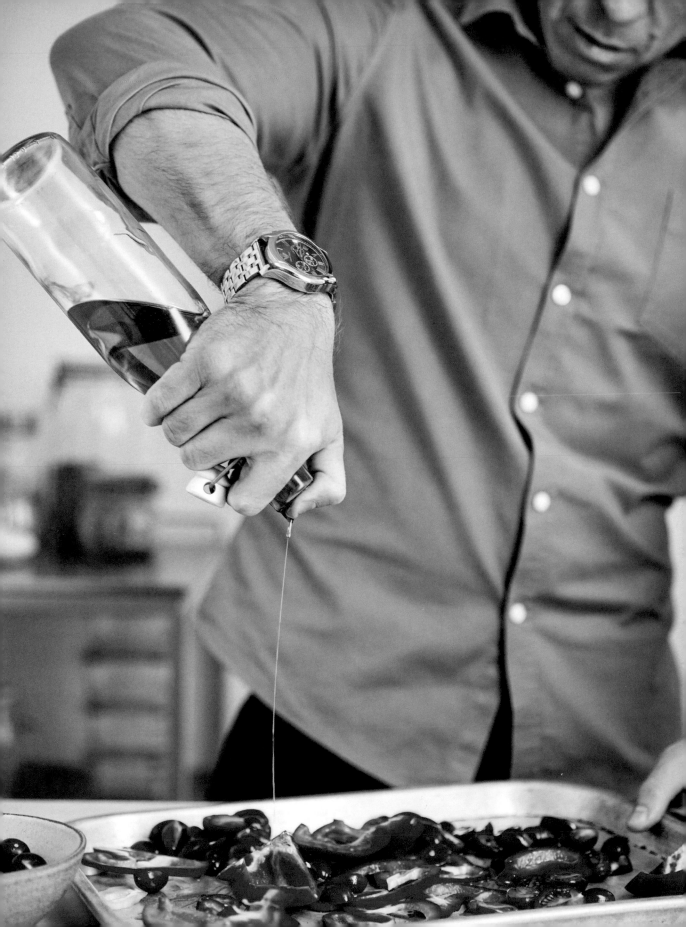

MY STORY

After years of trying and failing at all the usual diets, one day I realized that I needed to do something about the position I'd found myself in. I was seriously struggling with my weight and my health, both physical and mental, and these diets were costing me time and money but achieving nothing (put your hands up if you feel the same!). I really wanted to find a lifestyle which was sustainable for me. Whether you've found yourself in that same position or are only looking to shed a couple of pounds, I can guarantee you that meal prep is for you. As you'll discover when you read on, my old friend Frank inspired me with his cooking style and through him I discovered the joys of meal prepping. The rest is history, as they say.

Around 2003, when my weight reached 21st 6lb, I decided enough was enough and I couldn't carry on the way I was. I decided I'd go to my GP for help. The doctor told me that I was obese and gave me some anti-depressants to help with my mental health and a sheet of paper with a list of foods I could eat and another of foods I couldn't eat. I left the surgery in tears, shocked by what had happened. I was disappointed that I hadn't been given more support when it came to the fundamentals of food instead of simply being handed a box of anti-depressants and left to fend for myself.

I'm quite a proactive and practical person so I felt sure there had to be something else to try. Initially I did what many other people do, I signed up to the well-known diet plans, filled with promises that your weight will drop off you if you fast, count points or cut out food groups. I knew in my heart that this wasn't healthy but back then I felt it was all I had to turn to. After failing at many diets, including keto and cutting out carbs

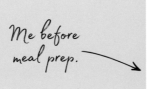

Me before meal prep.

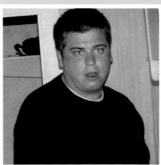

(which made me really ill), I remember thinking that this couldn't be sustainable for anyone at all and I had to find another way. I went to the library and read various books to try and educate myself as best I could. I'd seen plenty of people losing weight by restricting one food group or another, but then they'd regained all the weight, plus more, once they returned to eating normally. I knew from all the diets I'd tried that whatever I did had to be sustainable for me. A quick fix just wasn't an option.

As I'm a huge advocate for not wasting food, I will literally try and use everything. Eating excessively had been my downfall before, especially when I had a lack of basic knowledge about calories and what was and wasn't healthy. Now, though, I understood a great deal more about the nutritional value of food, so I knew that preparing my meals in advance was an absolute no-brainer for me. Meal prep meant I could eat what I wanted when I wanted, with the only restriction being the number of calories I was consuming across a whole day. I calculated the calories I could have by using a formula called TDEE (Total Daily Energy Expenditure, see page 35), depending on my weight-loss goals. Finally, I'd found the sustainable way of eating and lifestyle choice I'd been looking for. I don't call it a diet because I hate that word – it indicates something temporary that will come to an end, when in truth there is no end, as you have to eat for the rest of your life.

I initially got the idea of meal prepping from an old friend of mine called Frank. We lived together when I was a teenager and he became (and still is) a real inspiration to me in the kitchen. He always used to batch cook as money was tight at times, plus it was a fantastic way to ensure that nothing went to waste. He is now 82 years old and he still batch cooks to this day. (He's also the only man I know who's walked into a McDonald's and asked for egg, beans and chips with bread and butter on the side!)

Watching Frank batch cook over the years had really inspired me and now I knew I wanted to incorporate it into my everyday diet. I took the fundamentals of it and then added in more variety and organization. In my first four weeks of meal prepping, I lost around 12lb. I hadn't changed much about what I was eating, just the way in which I made meals, and of course my portion sizes. I'd met my new best friend: a set of kitchen scales, which I used to measure out my food. For the first time in a long time I was back in control of my weight and life. It was a great feeling!

I started using pen and paper to calculate calories by breaking down the macronutrients (macros), the protein, carbohydrate and fat, in each food. I found that tracking these things ensured my diet stayed balanced and the variety of nutrients I was consuming was vast. And I was shedding pounds of fat and loving life! I hadn't felt this confident in a very long time.

When I got down to 20 stone I decided to up my game and join a gym. Having lost a stone and a half thanks to my meal plan, I knew that I didn't need the gym to lose the weight but I knew it would help, not only physically but mentally as well. In the gym, I quickly acquired the nickname 'Fat John'. I wasn't overly concerned as I knew that in 12 months' time I'd be having the last laugh, and if anything it made me more determined to succeed.

The weight continued to fall off me. After around 6 months I was down to 17 stone. I'd seriously turned my life around and people at the gym would comment on how well I was looking. And I knew this was sustainable for life with or without the gym. I just had to adjust my daily calorie intake accordingly, if I was doing less exercise on a particular day. I was saving a fortune in cash, wasting no food and losing weight – it was great!

Twelve months later I was 12st 10lb and in the best shape of my life. I was no longer 'Fat John', I was now 'Slim John'! I was able to shop for clothes anywhere I wanted, often without even trying them on. As simple as it might sound, that was perhaps one of my greatest achievements. I no longer felt like a failure and it was an awesome feeling. Discovering how to eat what I wanted whilst feeling healthy was a light-bulb moment. I watched other people using restrictive diets and making themselves so unhappy whilst I was eating food that I really loved. My newfound tools allowed me to enjoy food all over again. It really is a powerful feeling when you realize it's not what you are eating that is the problem but instead the amount of calories you are consuming. I've used this meal prep approach ever since and haven't looked back once!

HOW I MET CHARLOTTE

Let's fast-forward to January 2017, when I met Charlotte online. Thanks to my weight loss, I was feeling better about myself, so I had the confidence to message her. We began speaking daily and I couldn't wait to meet her in person. For a while, Charlotte kept making excuses not to meet, but finally she agreed. I asked her if she'd like to go out for something to eat but she seemed extremely reluctant to go anywhere public. Not wanting to push her, I suggested we could have some food and drink at my house for our first date. I remember I wanted her to feel safe so I sent her a screenshot of a utility bill so her family would know where she was. I picked her up from her home in Blackpool and straight away I really liked her smile. Once we got chatting, I also liked who she was as a person, though I had no idea at this point how insecure she was about her appearance. When we first got back to mine, she sat down rather rigidly and still with her coat on, as if she was waiting for a bus, as my mum would say. But having already spoken at length before the date, we knew a lot about each other, so once we got past that initial awkwardness she relaxed and the date was a success.

After that evening, we kept in touch daily. Me being me, food was never too far from my mind so I'd sometimes ask inquisitively what she'd had for lunch or tea. I started to notice a pattern of her eating a very minimal amount of food and it often felt like she was making things up, saying that she'd eaten certain meals when in fact she hadn't eaten at all. I knew something was wrong as it was affecting her mood and her work, and her hair was falling out. I noticed the latter as there seemed to be black hair everywhere in my house and I made a joke to Charlotte about how it was going to blow up my Hoover. Sadly, I didn't realize at the time that I'd touched a nerve – but she was clearly insecure about it and, after doing some research, I learnt that the hair loss was due to a lack of the right nutrients.

As we became closer, Charlotte opened up to me about how she really felt. It turned out she hadn't been eating properly and was essentially starving herself in a last-ditch attempt to lose weight. I hadn't known Charlotte very long and it broke my heart to see how miserable she felt but I knew I could help change her life for the better because I'd been in such a similar situation myself.

I told Charlotte about my history with gaining weight and dieting and the nicknames I used to have to put up with. I showed her a pair of old jeans I'd kept as a reminder of my weight loss and so she realized I could truly empathize with how she was feeling. I then revealed how I'd changed my life and how I'd learnt to 'prep myself back to health'. Having shared all this with each other, we became even closer, but we were about to set off on an emotional weight-loss journey.

Together we discussed how I meal prepped. I explained that I cooked like this because it meant I could eat the food I loved, including burgers, pizzas and pasta, and I never felt hungry, plus I saved money and avoided food waste. Initially, Charlotte was rather sceptical, thinking it sounded too good to be true, but she saw the results I'd achieved so she decided to give it a shot. The first week we meal prepped together, Charlotte took her meal preps home with her and she was so impressed at the amount of effort, love and attention I'd put into the meals, she actually put a seatbelt around them for the journey back to Blackpool and sent me a picture as a joke!

As the pounds started falling off, Charlotte's smile got bigger and bigger and her confidence grew week on week – it was an absolute joy to watch. We eventually fell into a routine we enjoyed, and our love, respect and trust for each other grew weekly at a pace neither of us was expecting! I'm so glad we met each other. She's the best thing that's ever happened to me – and from what she tells me the feeling is mutual!

We now meal prep a full week's worth of meals on a Sunday and over time we have learnt so many tips and tricks, such as what freezes, what doesn't, what will last and what won't. It's made our lives so much easier, plus we waste hardly any food at all.

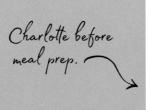

Charlotte before meal prep.

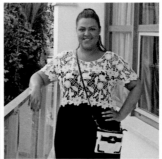

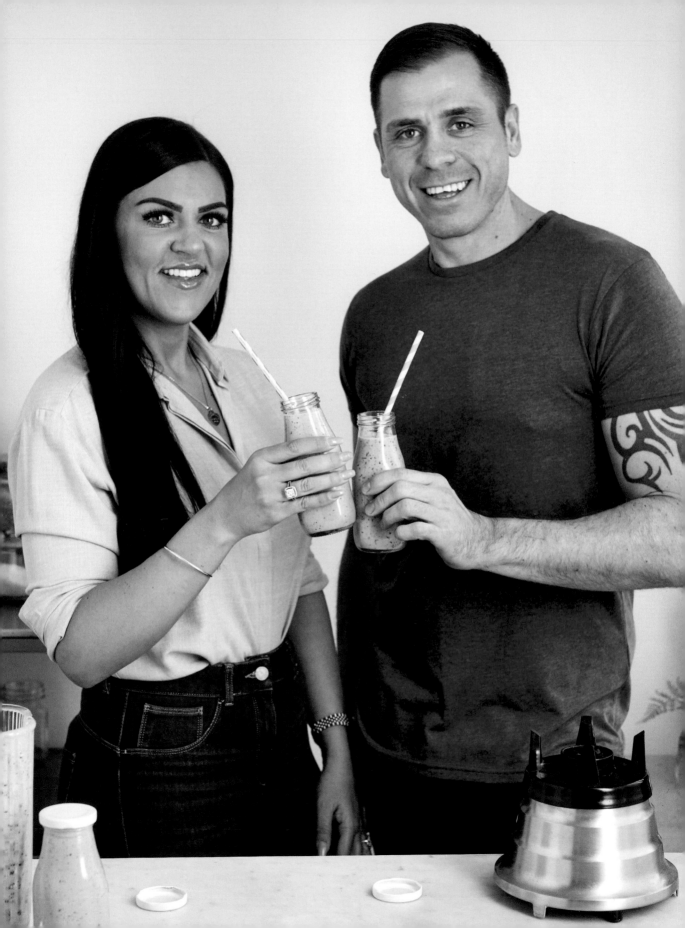

OUR MEAL PREP JOURNEY TOGETHER

The beauty of meal prepping is that it's entirely adaptable. We've tailored the concept to fit our current lifestyle, based around our time and commitments, which means you can use this book however works best for your life, though obviously the fundamentals stay the same.

We started looking in the fridge and freezer on a Friday night when Charlotte came to my house after work, figuring out what would go off soon if not cooked. Then we would write a list of additional ingredients which would work alongside the food we already had. On a Saturday we'd shop and search for bargains at local markets, supermarkets and online. Then on Sundays we'd cook. Some weeks we would cook a wide array of batch meals, aiming for variety; other weeks we focused on cost, often managing to spend less than 60p per meal. Other times we focused on trying out new and exciting ideas. Together we calculated what Charlotte's calories should be for any given day/week based on her age, activity levels, job, etc. so we could devise a plan of action especially for her. And so, Sunday meal prep was born.

Week by week, we dedicated our Sundays to prepping our meals and Charlotte started to see the pounds drop off her – just as they had done for me many years earlier. I remember when Charlotte had lost about 2 stone: you could see the glow in her face, she was gaining confidence and was wearing clothes she'd only ever dreamed of wearing. She too had a wardrobe full of black clothes as I once did, and her wardrobe looks so different today, just like mine does. I fell in love with Charlotte because of how sincere she is, and how caring of others, and above all our ability to work together and support each other in things so strongly. For the first time in my life I wanted more for someone else than for myself – I'd never loved someone as much as I love her. Call it a cliché but it's the God's honest truth.

Charlotte and I continued on our meal prep journey together and I began posting about it on Instagram. People seemed interested in my posts and I gained a few followers. I had started losing weight before the era of social media and influencers, so I hadn't been swayed by any of the misconceptions and trends which have taken hold online but which not only aren't useful for weight loss but can in fact be dangerous. I was posting about my meal prep from a genuine place and based on my real-life success, and it really seemed to resonate with my followers. I didn't know much about Instagram, but I was getting messages from people all over the world about how we'd inspired them, and it made me think that maybe we could actually help people, all from my little kitchen and with just an iPhone. So I made an effort to post weekly. The feedback I was getting was amazing. I was starting to receive messages from people telling me about the weight they were losing, and thanking me and Charlotte for the inspiration we'd given them. I was amazed at how the little we did seemed to be having a big impact; it was incredible and just fuelled us further.

Christmas 2017 was fast approaching and Charlotte was nearly at her goal weight of 9st 10lb, all without even stepping into a gym. Charlotte's friends, family and work colleagues had all seen her amazing transformation and were constantly asking her what diet she was on. Charlotte would take her meal preps to work, and soon she had colleagues dropping into her office at lunchtime just to see what she'd brought in to eat that day! As we were eating such a huge variety of food, a lot of her friends and family liked the look of it and started to follow me on Instagram, keen to try it for themselves. Many of them were ditching conventional diet plans, inspired by Charlotte's new-found love of food, freedom and fashion, a lifestyle she'd adopted with me. Many of them now swear by meal prep too!

At this point I knew we could help many more people achieve results like ours. We were getting more and more positive feedback online. It became part of our weekly routine to post tips, tricks and updates on Sunday evenings. Soon we saw people saying, 'Does anyone else sit glued to Instagram on Sunday evenings to see what they've made?!' We tried our best to take good photographs to post for our eager followers but our only kit was an iPhone and the kitchen light bulb. With the daylight disappearing into dusk, the limited lighting meant our pictures could sometimes be hard to make out so I would often ask Charlotte to stand on a chair in the kitchen, holding up a baking tray wrapped in tin foil in an attempt to reflect more light on to the meals on the worktop. A battle of wills would ensue as Charlotte complained that her arms were hurting whilst I tried to ensure we got the perfect shot!

One day a parcel arrived at my house addressed to The Meal Prep King. I was confused – no one had ever sent me a parcel using my Instagram name before. I opened it and inside was a professional photography light. Since there was no sender's name on the parcel, I said to Charlotte, 'You'll never guess what someone's sent me!' I didn't twig that it was Charlotte who had sent it to me until she said, 'Who do you think has sent it to you, John?' That's when the penny dropped and I realized she really didn't like holding our makeshift tin-foil light reflector!

Although we've been doing all this for some time now, it just doesn't get boring to us. We absolutely love shopping together for ingredients and look forward to it rather than seeing it as a chore. Going to local markets and supermarkets is like a day out, allowing us to spend quality time together which we otherwise wouldn't have. We still meal prep each Sunday, and at the end of the prepping day we take photographs to post on Instagram. What started out as something to help Charlotte has ended up bringing us closer together and turned into something we both enjoy. Collectively we've lost 15 stone and have gained a lot more than just falling in love with each other. Couples who meal prep together stay together!

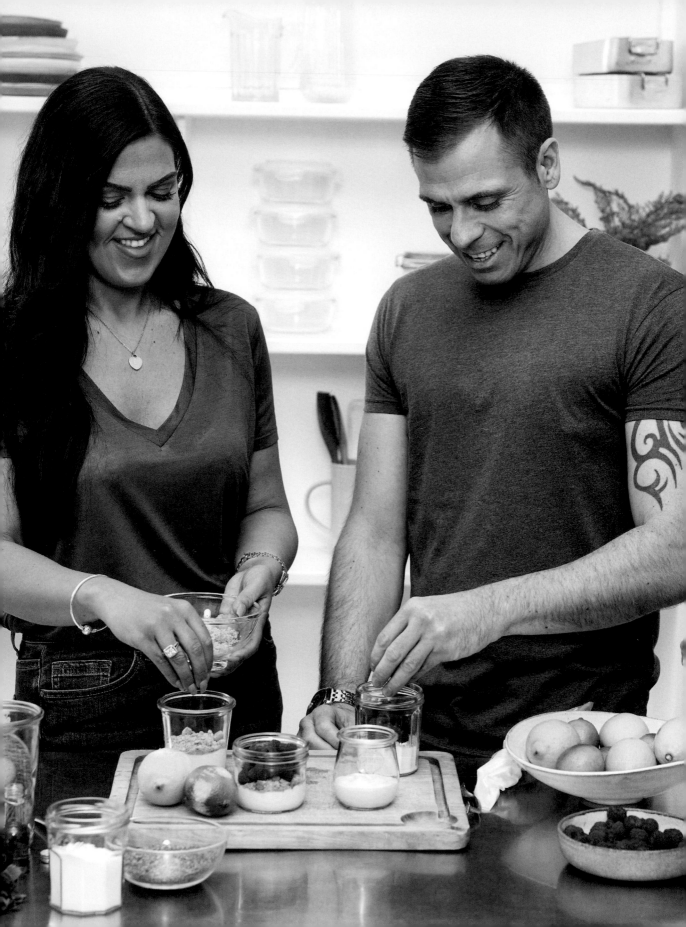

MEAL PREP IS FOR EVERYONE

It doesn't matter what you're doing or where you are, you can meal prep. Over the years I've heard all the excuses under the sun, so I'm here to show you that you can follow this plan whether you're a student living in a shared house or cooking for a big family. Once you start meal prepping and realize how much time and money you're saving, you won't ever look back!

Meal prepping is incredibly versatile and can be completely tailored to your lifestyle. Charlotte and I meal prep to fit around our commitments but we know some people who meal prep four weeks in advance and others who prep three days in advance. We both work full time and we live separately, so we meal prep when we see each other at the weekends; it's one of the many things which brings us closer. Figure out when works best for you to do your meal prep and what time you like to eat your meals, then you're all set. You might find it easier to meal prep on a Monday evening, over the course of a couple of evenings, during the day or over the weekend – try it out and find your ideal meal prep time! This is the joy of meal prepping: it's entirely flexible and can be personalized to everyone's tastes, budget and requirements.

When it comes to eating out and going on holidays, don't be afraid to eat food that you haven't meal prepped yourself. If you start to overcomplicate things by calorie counting on special occasions or always bringing your own meal prep in your bag, then you'll take the enjoyment out of food, which is exactly what we want to avoid. If I went to a restaurant and started calorie counting my meal, that would be taking it too far. Life is about balance, so enjoy that dinner out guilt free!

People often ask me how I stay on track constantly. The simple answer is that I don't, and the chances are neither will you. Do you know why? Because you're only human! However, not staying on track isn't a reason to give up, far from it. Pick yourself up afterwards, don't blame yourself or beat yourself up because you think you've failed, just get back on track. Make some healthier choices, and don't be too hard on yourself. Remember, success is about what you do consistently, not what you do now and again, so repeat the behaviour you're aiming for as often as you can and soon it will become second nature.

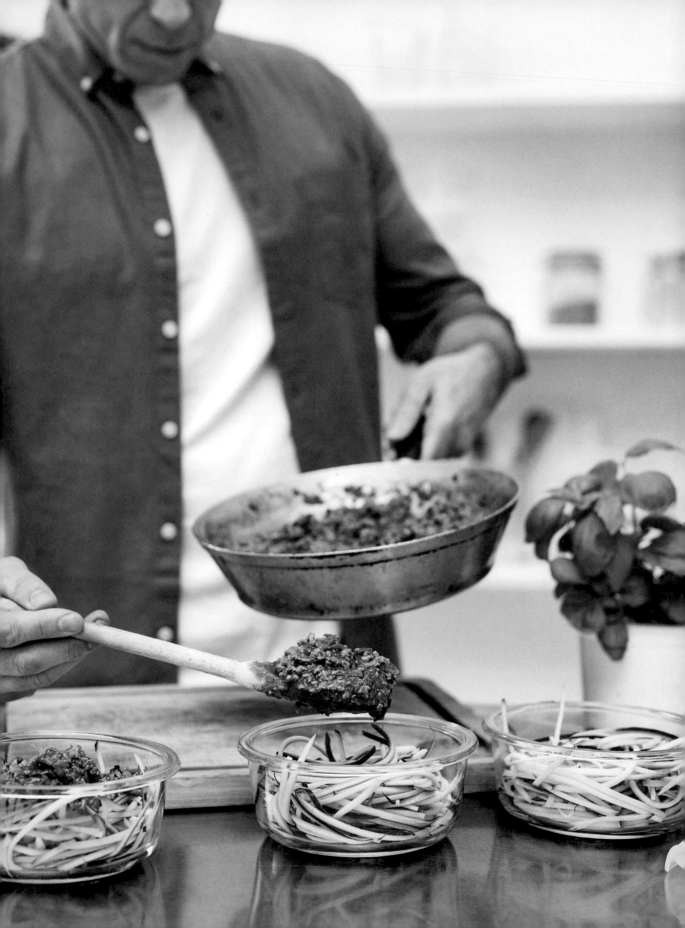

JOHN AND CHARLOTTE'S RULES FOR MEAL PREP SUCCESS

Check out our top ten tips that will get you well on your way to becoming a meal prep king or queen:

1 SHOP AROUND: You'll be amazed at some of the deals you can find. We often shop at supermarkets late at night as they are much quieter. You also find the odd gem marked down in price, often as much as 70 per cent off, if you shop towards the end of the day, so make sure you have a look in the reduced section.

2 USE LOCAL MARKETS: I realize that not everyone has a local market but it's well worth the effort if you can find one, even if you have to go out of your way to get there. We tend to go to Bury Market in Manchester, and we make a day out of it and turn it into a little adventure. We have picked up some absolute bargains there, including 3kg of blueberries for £1.50, which would have cost us about £40 in a supermarket.

3 LOOK AT WHAT YOU'VE ALREADY GOT IN THE FRIDGE: Look for items getting close to their use-by or best-before dates and focus on those to create your meals; you'll be amazed at some of the creations you can come up with. Don't be afraid to use things that are past their best-before date – these are often fine beyond the stated shelf life, just check they still look all right and use your common sense.

However, use-by dates are not the same as best-before dates. Never use items past their stated use-by date.

4 DON'T BE AFRAID OF FAILURE: Just because you make a mistake with a recipe or you're not happy with how your meal prep turns out one day, please don't give up. Over the years I've done all the things you shouldn't do when it comes to cooking, including burning food and serving Charlotte some pretty inedible meals. Making mistakes is how we learn, so embrace them.

5 BE ORGANIZED: Once you have decided which days to allocate for your meal prepping, plan your menu the day before to ensure you have everything you're going to need in advance. That way you don't have any excuses to skip meal prep or give up before you've finished. This is a no-brainer but make a list before you go shopping as it saves on time and stops you buying things you don't actually need. Charlotte sometimes forgets the shopping list (quite often, truth be told!) so rather than go back and get it, we see if we can do the full shop without forgetting anything. When we get back, we check to see how close we were to the list we left behind. If we have forgotten anything, one of us will nip to the shops quickly, though we try to avoid this if we can – and sometimes this leads to us adapting our menu and coming up with new meals!

6 **VARIATION IS KEY:** Variety keeps things interesting and means you are less likely to get bored and give up on what is essential to your new lifestyle. Try and mix things up as much as possible!

7 **WEIGH EVERYTHING:** Well, almost everything! This is one of the key ways to keep your calories on track, especially if you are new to meal prep. People are often shocked at how many calories are in foods once they start weighing them out. I think this is a fundamental way to learn about calories and portion control as it helps you to be more aware of the calorie content of food, plus you'll get used to seeing how much food you should have on your plate visually (for example, a healthy portion of pasta is about the size of a tennis ball). A good little set of kitchen scales is an invaluable and inexpensive meal prep tool and one which can help guarantee success.

8 **USE GOOD-QUALITY MEAL PREP CONTAINERS:** There is nothing worse than meal prep containers that leak, so make sure you choose the right meal prep tub for you. Glass can be heavy to carry about, so it's best kept for food you'll be eating at home, and if you have multiple glass containers they generally don't stack well so storage can become difficult. Stainless steel containers are fantastic and lighter than glass ones. You can recycle old glass jars for salad

dressings. Try and find yourself a good-quality plastic range you can reuse for many years – the ones I currently use are three years old. If you ever want to invest in a new set, you can upcycle the old ones by using them as storage containers for dry ingredients and spices in your cupboard. I'm currently developing my own range of containers, so keep an eye on my website (www.themealprepking.com) for when these become available.

9 **MAKE YOUR OWN VERSIONS OF YOUR GUILTY PLEASURES:** For me this is really important as it allows you to save on calories, because you know exactly what has gone into your meal, and enables you to eat more of other foods. By doing this, you're setting yourself up for long-term success. For example, on page 203, you'll find my own version of a double chocolate doughnut. At only 120 calories each they allow you to enjoy something which would otherwise be very high in calories, making room for more food in your daily allowance. And who doesn't want to eat more food?

10 **ENJOY WHAT YOU'RE DOING:** This is vital. Make sure you create a system which you enjoy so that meal prep can become a sustainable way of life. Don't think of meal prep as a diet but rather a change in lifestyle that will help you for the rest of your life.

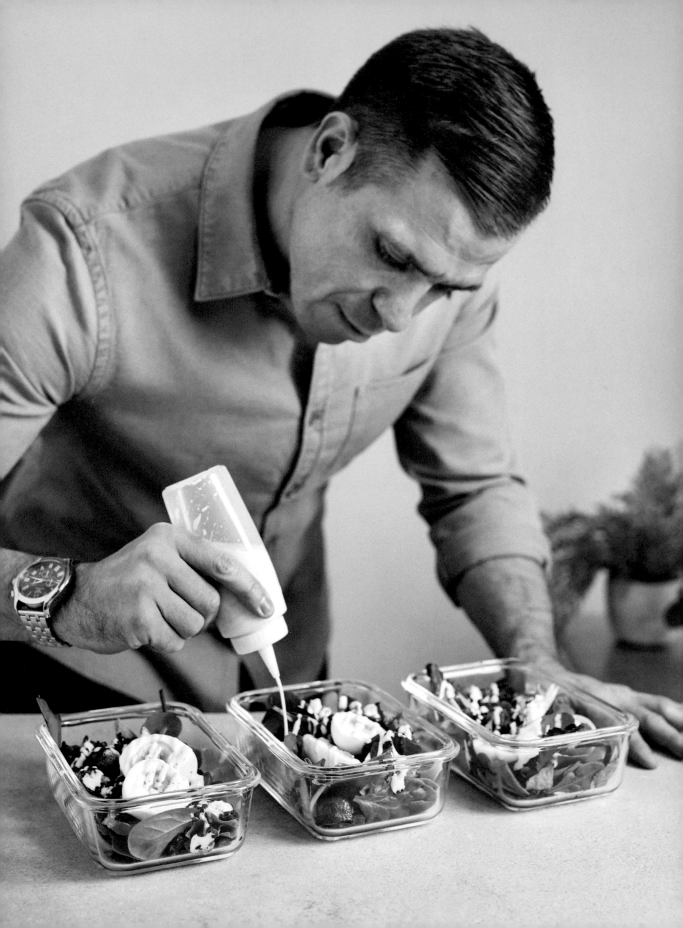

HOW TO DO THE 21-DAY PLAN

Firstly, congratulations on embarking on this 21-day meal prep plan. This is the first step towards a happy, healthier you. Why 21 days? I hear you ask. Many years ago I read that it takes 21 days to make or break a habit. Obviously it's much easier to make a habit than it is to break an old one, and this is why I ballooned in weight – it was easier for me to overeat than to stop. The key thing to breaking habits is consistency, so focusing on what you're eating over the next three weeks will give you a much better chance of success with losing weight, keeping it off, and saving money and time. I've been doing it for 18 years now and have never looked back.

Meal prepping is so adaptable and can fit any lifestyle, so I didn't want this plan to be too prescriptive. You can do what works best for you. Over the next few pages you'll find out what you need to get you started, as well as example menus for the full three weeks of meal prep. You can either follow this plan to the letter or simply swap out recipes for other ones you prefer.

'The key to breaking habits is consistency'

GETTING STARTED

Before you embark on the 21-day plan, here are a few things to get you well on your way, from storage containers to the essential ingredients you'll need in your cupboard. Read on to learn everything you need to know about meal prepping so that you can see the transformation you want in your body.

Storage

It goes without saying that storage is one of the key things to get right when it comes to meal prep. Without containers, you won't have any way to store your pre-prepared meals, so they're the first thing you need to sort out. I highly recommend square or rectangular ones as circular containers don't stack as well and take up more space. There are so many advantages to good containers: you can reuse them, you can freeze them, you can label them and they're incredibly durable if you get good ones (glass or stainless-steel ones are the best for this). I get many questions about storage so have given some answers below to ensure you store your meals in the best way you can:

★ **How long will meals last?**
Meals will last perfectly fine for up to three days in the fridge. Aim to get your prepared food into the fridge within 60–90 minutes of cooking. Take any food out of a hot pan and away from any heat source so that it's not being kept warm by the residual heat. Do not leave food out for hours or – worse – overnight. This is a big no-no!

★ **Do I need to cool the food before storing?**
All food needs to be cooled quickly and thoroughly before it is put in the fridge or freezer. If you don't do this, you run the risk of increasing the temperature in your fridge or freezer and creating an environment where bacteria will multiply. This could affect the shelf life of your prepped meals as well as other foods stored in there. Some top tips of mine are to cool rice and pasta under cold running water after cooking to speed up the cooling time and to stir food regularly whilst it is

cooling down, which will help it cool more evenly. You can also spread some foods over a larger area, such as on a large plate, to help them cool more quickly.

★ **What temperature should my fridge be at?**
Your fridge should always remain below 5°C for it to keep food at its optimum.

★ **What do I do when the weather is hot and I want to take my meal prep out with me?**
A cool bag with ice packs is a must! That way you never miss out on meal prep and your food stays safe.

★ **How do I store the sauces that go with the meal prep?**
Store things like gravy, coleslaw and other sauces in a separate small container which fits inside the meal prep tub to keep the food fresher and avoid it going soggy. For some meals, the sauce is supposed to be served cold so storing it in a little pot means you can simply remove it from the container before reheating your meal and then pour on the sauce after.

Freezing

Your freezer is your best friend and, with time, you'll become a bit of an expert in how to use it to its full potential. I appreciate that the amount of available freezer space will vary from person to person, however, using the space you have to your advantage can be a useful meal prep tool. Freezing is also a great way of limiting any food waste.

Of course, freezing food takes a bit of practice as not everything freezes equally well in terms of keeping its quality, as I've discovered over the years. I want to impart my wisdom so you can avoid making the same mistakes I have! I've also included a freezer logo next to the recipes that freeze well, so that you can see this at a glance. Not all my meals can be frozen though, and that's okay; just make sure you eat those ones first, within three days of cooking.

Freezing tips:

★ Food should be frozen on the day it's made.

★ Freezer bags can be a great way to store things like soups, rice, even bread. They can be stored flat, and they are extremely cheap – so they can be a great alternative to buying meal prep tubs should you want to keep costs down even further. You can reuse them as well, so make sure you wash them out after you've reheated your meal and save them for future meals.

★ If a particular dish has salad with it, simply freeze it without the salad and add fresh salad when you defrost the meal.

Reheating

How you reheat food is key to staying healthy and making sure that you can enjoy your meal prep as much as possible. Nobody wants to get ill!

★ If a meal for the next day is frozen, take it out of the freezer the night before and defrost it in the fridge. The meal should be thoroughly defrosted before reheating.

★ Reheat food until piping hot throughout. If you're using a microwave, remember they don't heat evenly, so take your food out halfway through the cooking time and give it a stir before continuing.

★ All foods should be reheated until they reach and maintain 70°C or above for 2 minutes.

★ Foods like soup can be reheated in a pan instead of in a microwave.

★ Never reheat your meal preps more than once. Equally, don't refreeze them once they're defrosted because the more times you cool and reheat food, the higher the risk of food poisoning. Bacteria can multiply when food is cooled too slowly and won't be killed if the food is reheated insufficiently.

★ Top tip: sprinkle rice with a little water before reheating as this will stop it becoming too dry.

How to plan

The best way to plan your meals is to first go through your fridge and freezer to see what you already have. This is a fantastic way of saving money, and using up what you already have avoids food waste. It's a great way to start planning your meal prep menu – don't be afraid to experiment with your ingredients, you might create a new favourite meal! Once we've got our list sorted, we head to the supermarket and the local market to snap up the best deals. Whilst using a shopping list saves money and time, it also means there's no excuse not to make the meals as you will have all the ingredients.

By planning your shopping and your meals ahead, you won't find yourself with a trolley full of unhealthy snacks and random ingredients, and you will stick to your budget as well. Not only this but by prepping your meals in advance you'll have more free time to do the things you really enjoy.

Kit basics

To get yourself on the road to becoming a meal prep king or queen, there are a few essential bits of kit and ingredients you'll need in your kitchen. The recipes in this book don't require any fancy equipment and I've listed the key kit basics you'll need to get you meal prepping in no time:

• Meal prep containers
• Scales – digital are more accurate but analogue ones are also fine
• Non-stick frying pan
• Saucepan
• Cast-iron griddle pan
• Food processor
• Baking tray
• Chopping boards
• Spatulas and spoons
• Chef's knife
• Measuring jug
• Doughnut tray

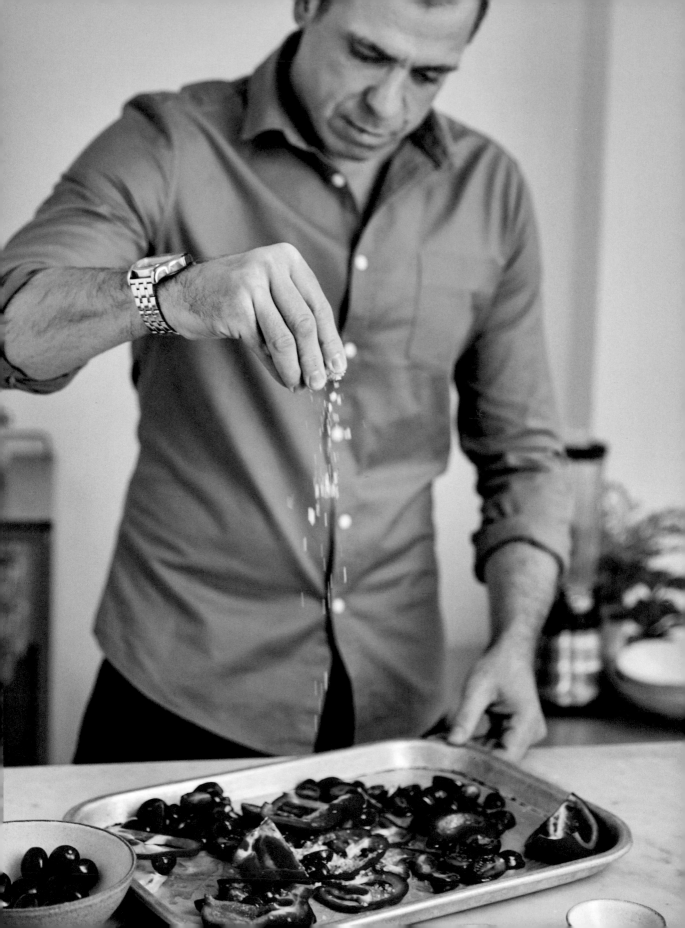

Cupboard essentials

Having these cupboard essentials in the house will make meal prep a doddle, and making the best of them will make your life easier as well. They'll also be there to cook something healthy with if you ever find yourself without meals in the fridge or freezer. To keep costs down, always check what you have in the cupboard, along with the fridge, before planning your meal prep.

Don't rush out and get them all at once. Instead, build them up over time as you work your way through the recipes and find a meal prep routine that works for you.

Fridge
- bag of fresh salad
- bag of fresh spinach (frozen works just as well)
- butter

General
- baking powder
- balsamic vinegar
- bicarbonate of soda
- brown rice
- brown sugar
- caster sugar
- flour: self-raising, plain and wholemeal
- honey
- lentils (tinned green ones and dry red lentils)
- oats
- salt and pepper
- soy sauce
- stock cubes (vegetable, chicken and beef)
- sweetener
- tomato purée
- vanilla extract
- white rice
- Worcestershire sauce

Tinned goods
- butter beans
- chickpeas
- coconut milk
- tomatoes

Oils
- coconut oil
- low-cal spray oil
- olive oil
- sesame oil
- vegetable oil

Spices and herbs
- allspice
- bay leaves
- cayenne pepper
- chilli powder
- Chinese five-spice powder
- curry powder
- fennel seeds
- garam masala
- garlic powder
- garlic salt
- ground cinnamon
- ground coriander
- ground cumin
- ground nutmeg
- ground turmeric
- mixed herbs
- mustard powder
- nigella seeds
- onion granules
- onion salt
- oregano
- paprika
- smoked paprika

Spice mixes

People assume spices are all about heat when in fact they're delicious flavour enhancers that can completely elevate the simplest of recipes to a tasty dish. The truth is spice mixes don't have to be hot. Though the ones listed have a little bit of a kick to them (which you can adjust to your own taste), it doesn't always have to be the case. There are many examples in this book alone, from the turmeric chicken on page 110 to the smoky paprika popcorn on page 205, which aren't spicy at all.

Spices have been an integral part of my weight loss and how I sustain it as they're a great way of keeping food fresh and exciting without adding lots of calories. People have this preconceived idea that meal prep and diet foods have to be bland in order to help you lose weight. I myself thought this when I was following other diets, until I discovered that spices can add different levels of flavour and texture to dishes. Since then, I've been learning more about them and experimenting with my own blends that I want to share with you. Spices are a great way to liven up your meals, so experiment yourself and create some absolutely delicious mouth-watering meals. Not only do spices enhance the flavour but they also give your dishes a vibrant colour, which will make them more appealing to eat (not that you'll have any problem with the recipes in this book!). It's amazing what you can create in the comfort of your own home.

In the cupboard essentials section on page 31, you'll see a list of some of the basic spices I recommend you keep to hand. This section builds on that, so you can learn how to create spice mixes yourself instead of buying pre-made ones in the shops. You can also tweak them according to your own taste (I love heat in my recipes so I always add a little extra chilli wherever I can). Don't rush out and buy the ingredients all at once: slowly build up your spice cupboard over time as you explore the different recipes within the book.

Each of these recipes makes more spice mix than you'll need to make the meals in this book but you can store the rest in an airtight container to use later.

Shawarma mix

4 tsp ground cumin
4 tsp ground coriander
4 tsp paprika
2 tsp ground turmeric
1 tsp cayenne pepper
a pinch of ground
   cinnamon
1 tsp garlic powder
salt and pepper

Peri peri seasoning

4 tsp paprika
2 tsp onion powder
2 tsp garlic powder
2 tsp ground cardamom
1 tsp ground ginger
1/2 tsp caster sugar
2 tsp dried oregano
1 tsp cayenne pepper
salt and pepper

Fajita seasoning

1 tsp chilli powder
   (adjust according to
   your heat tolerance)
1 tbsp smoked paprika
a pinch of ground cumin
1 tsp garlic powder
1 tsp dried oregano
a pinch of onion powder
a pinch of cayenne
   pepper

Cajun seasoning

2 tbsp paprika
1 tbsp garlic powder
1 tsp ground black pepper
1 tsp ground white pepper
1/2 tsp onion powder
1/2 tsp dried oregano
1/2 tsp cayenne pepper
a pinch of dried thyme
a pinch of salt

Jerk seasoning

1 tsp garlic powder
1 tsp cayenne pepper
1 tsp onion powder
1/2 tsp dried thyme
1/2 tsp dried parsley
1/2 tsp paprika
1/4 tsp allspice
a pinch of crushed dried
   red pepper
a pinch of ground
   cinnamon
salt and pepper

Chilli spice mix

1/2 tsp chilli powder
   (adjust the amount
   according to your heat
   tolerance)
1 tsp smoked paprika
1/2 tsp ground cumin
1/2 tsp garlic powder
1/2 tsp dried oregano
1/2 tsp ground coriander
1/2 tsp black pepper
1/2 tsp ground fenugreek

Thai spice mix

1 tsp ground cumin
1 tsp lemon pepper
1 tsp chilli powder
1 tsp garlic powder
2 tsp ground ginger
1 tsp onion powder
salt and pepper

Harissa seasoning

2 tsp smoked paprika
1 tsp ground cumin
1 tsp ground coriander
1 tsp chilli powder
a pinch of sea salt
1 tsp garlic powder
1/2 tsp dried mint

Curry powder

2 tsp ground turmeric
2 tsp ground coriander
a large pinch of chilli
   powder
1 tsp ground cumin
2 tsp smoked paprika
1 tsp onion salt

Mexican seasoning

1 tsp chilli powder
1/2 tsp garlic powder
1/2 tsp dried oregano
1 tsp paprika
1 1/2 tsp ground cumin

How to calculate your daily calorie allowance

Now that you know how to store your meal prep and what kit you need in your kitchen, the next step is to calculate how many calories you can have a day. This is key to the plan: by taking in fewer calories from food and drink than you burn through your daily activity you'll lose weight. Many diets restrict your intake of one nutrient, such as carbohydrate or fat, but scientific studies show that when it comes to weight loss, it's simply calories that count (although of course eating a good balance of nutrients is important for health). Provided you eat fewer calories than you burn, you will lose weight – it's a pretty simple concept! The key to long-term success is to find a plan that you can comfortably live with rather than embarking on strict diets that are hard to maintain, which is why meal prep is so sustainable. It's not a diet but a lifestyle.

Read on to learn how to calculate how many calories you can consume a day:

'The key to long-term success is to find a plan that you can comfortably live with'

1. Find your Total Daily Energy Expenditure (TDEE)

TDEE is an estimate of how many calories you burn each day. It is calculated by first estimating your Basal Metabolic Rate (BMR), then multiplying that value by an activity multiplier. Your BMR is an estimate of how many calories your body burns at rest. The best way to calculate your BMR is to use an online calculator. But if you want to do it the old-fashioned way, use the most popular equation (Mifflin-St Jeor) and punch in the numbers:

Men: 10 x weight (kg) + 6.25 x height (cm) – 5 x age (years) + 5

Women: 10 x weight (kg) + 6.25 x height (cm) – 5 x age (years) – 161

Now multiply your BMR figure by your Physical Activity Level (PAL), which is a rough measure of your lifestyle activity (choose the figure that most fits your level of activity from the table below).

PHYSICAL ACTIVITY LEVEL (PAL)	MULTIPLIER	DESCRIPTION
Mostly inactive	1.2	Mainly sitting
Fairly active	1.3	Sitting, some walking, exercise once or twice per week
Moderately active	1.4	Regular walking, or exercise two to three times per week
Active	1.5	Exercise or sport more than three times per week
Very active	1.7	Physically active job or intense daily exercise or sport

2. Count the calories in the food you consume

Your TDEE will give you a good estimate of the number of calories you require each day to keep your weight steady. To lose weight, you will need to consume fewer calories than your TDEE. As a rule of thumb, a calorie deficit of 500 cals per day should result in a 0.5kg (1lb) weight loss per week. This can be achieved either through consuming 500 fewer calories, burning 500 more calories, or a combination of the two. The easiest way to track calories consumed is with an app and there are lots of them available, so find the one which works best for you.

All the meals in this plan provide less than 500 cals so you will easily be able to tally the calorie counts for each recipe and check that the overall total is about 500 less than your TDEE (those with higher TDEE will require more snacks). We suggest you have one breakfast and two main meals each day, plus one or more snacks, depending on your TDEE.

Exercise

Doing exercise is fantastic for your wellbeing, including your mental health, besides the obvious benefit that it will speed up your weight loss. However, exercising isn't essential for success on this plan – it all comes down to your free time and availability. Charlotte lost 6 stone in 10 months without going to the gym and only felt confident to go into a gym once she'd done so. Everyone is completely different and how you incorporate exercise into this plan is completely flexible.

Charlotte and I love walking to the point that if we're really craving a chocolate bar we'll walk two miles to the shop to get it and then walk the two miles back so we've earnt it. So if you can walk somewhere instead of driving or taking the bus, that's an easy way to squeeze in a bit of exercise. If you can't afford to join a gym or just don't feel it's for you, then home workouts are another great solution: there are loads on YouTube or you could download a workout app. The main thing is finding something you enjoy and can fit into your everyday life.

Things to watch out for in your diet

There's nothing you can't eat when it comes to my meal prep plan, as it's all about common sense and moderation! No food groups are cut out and this is one of the reasons why I've been meal prepping for so long. I just cannot stand restrictive eating – you feel obliged to remove certain things from your diet and guilty if you don't. I do drink alcohol but I limit my intake, just as I do for caffeine, but don't feel that you have to remove anything from your diet, because you really don't. However, educated choices will help allow you to consume more food for the same amount of calories. Remember, this is ideally going to be something you do for the rest of your life so it has to be sustainable for you.

There is only one thing I advise you to avoid and that's trans fats, as they increase levels of blood cholesterol and raise your risk of heart disease. To reduce your intake, make sure you read labels and check ingredients lists for partially hydrogenated oil. Although some trans fat is found naturally in animal products, it's artificial trans fat you need to be careful of. Thankfully, these are far less common than they were a few years ago but may be found in certain hard margarines, pastries, biscuits, snacks, takeaways and fast foods.

I would suggest you add more fibre into your diet as it's so good for your gut health. It feeds the trillions of microbes that live in your gut and influence your mood, appetite, weight and so much more. Some foods high in fibre are wholegrain breakfast cereals, porridge oats, wholegrain breads, bulgur wheat and things like brown rice and wholemeal pasta. Try adding lentils and beans to stews to add extra fibre as well as bulking them up. Also, adding more fresh fruit and vegetables such as oranges, bananas, apples and strawberries, broccoli, sweetcorn and carrots (a few of my favourites!) to your diet will help boost your fibre intake as well as giving you a whole range of other important nutrients. Plus, extra fibre also helps keep you feeling full for longer, which is always a positive.

I've listed some of my favourite foods below so you can add them to your diet, too, if you want to:

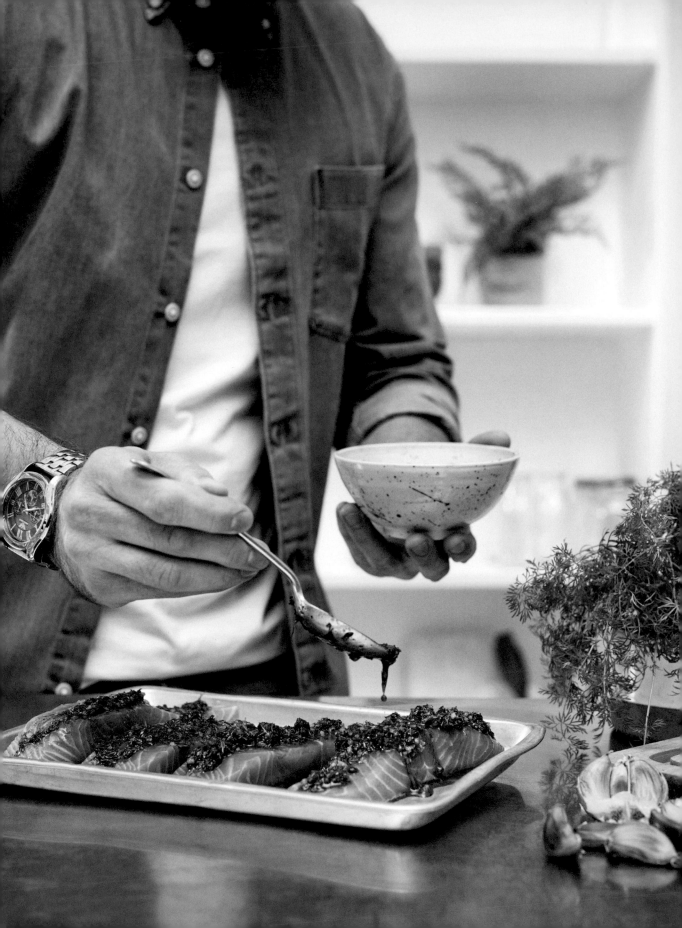

★ **Spinach:** I add spinach to everything! Recently I bought some spinach and its use-by date was the next day. As you know, I hate food waste so I made sure we had it in everything: roast dinner with spinach, eggs with spinach, and I even thought about putting it in porridge but Charlotte drew the line at that one . . .

★ **Honey:** it's such a fantastic natural sweetener and we love the stuff! It is important to remember that it does contain a lot of calories, but it can still be enjoyed in moderation as a substitute for refined sugar or syrup.

★ **Porridge oats:** these are an absolute favourite in our house as they're inexpensive, versatile and tasty. From protein bars and overnight oats to being blitzed up and used as flour, oats can be included in your diet in a variety of ways. In addition, oats are filling and will help you stay fuller for longer.

★ **Tinned tomatoes:** they have so many uses – I would be here all day if I had to list them all. Naturally low in calories, they make a fantastic base for things like curries, casseroles, chilli con carne and much more. Plus they're cheap as chips!

THE 21-DAY PLAN

To get you started with meal prepping, I've drawn up a 3-week plan to help you see exactly how your weeks might look and also how much variety you can get into your diet, as I'm a big fan of packing in as many nutrients as possible. As I mentioned earlier, they say it takes 21 days to form a new habit, so if you can smash this 3-week plan, then you are set for the future. If you're someone who likes to follow a plan, you can stick to this one closely, or if you want to switch things up, you'll find empty grids on pages 55–7 which you can fill in with the recipes of your choice. The plan will feed one person so just double it up for two people or quadruple it for four (or you can double it up if it's just you who's doing the plan and freeze the meals for later).

Charlotte and I do all our meal prep on Sundays, which takes us 7 to 8 hours, but I'm aware that that would be a very intensive meal prepping session for anyone just starting out. So for this beginner's plan I've suggested you do a session on a Sunday and then do another batch of cooking on Wednesday evening. Of course, it doesn't have to be restricted to these days at all. Meal prep is entirely adaptable to your lifestyle so you can find a time – or times – which works best for you and your schedule. You might want to split it up over a couple of evenings or you might only want to batch cook for the next two days – it's up to you!

The day before your first meal prep session you'll need a shopping list. If you're following this plan to the letter, then you'll find the relevant lists on the upcoming pages so you can easily take a photo of them before you hit the shops or the market. You might already have some of the ingredients, so be sure to check the fridge and cupboards before you go shopping to avoid waste and save yourself money. When we get home from the shops we freeze any of the perishables that aren't going to be used straight away and defrost them later on in the week when we need them – this way you avoid having to go to the shops multiple times. Breakfast and snacks can be made very quickly.

I would also suggest that you have a clear-out of your freezer ahead of meal prepping to make sure that you have enough space to store everything. We're all guilty of having too many half-eaten bags of frozen peas in the freezer! You might find forgotten food in there which you can incorporate into your meal plan to make sure that you avoid any food waste. The longer you meal prep, the easier it will become as your freezer fills up with tasty meals that you can defrost at a later date, so having enough space is key. Sometimes life will get in the way but if you have some frozen meals ready to go, you won't have any excuse to slip up. Let your freezer become your friend!

'If you can smash this 3-week plan, then you are set for the future'

WEEK 1

The first week of meal prepping is always the most labour-intensive week as you're starting from scratch, slowly building up the meals you have in your freezer and getting used to meal prep itself. Once you've got this first week out of the way, you'll be well on your way for the rest of the 21-day plan with a lot of ready-made meals in the freezer.

To make on the *first* meal prep day:
- ★ banana and blueberry miniature loaves (makes 10, freeze 9)
- ★ jacket potato with pork and BBQ beans
- ★ butter bean and vegetable biryani (double quantity – freeze 2 of the 4 portions)
- ★ turmeric chicken with rice and greens
- ★ garlic chicken and kale spaghetti
- ★ beetroot hummus, protein balls (makes 10, freeze 8)
- ★ homemade granola

To make on the *second* meal prep day:
- ★ super green soup (double quantity – freeze 2 of the 4 portions)
- ★ full English breakfast wrap (makes 4, freeze 3)
- ★ fridge forage vegetable and lentil bowls
- ★ harissa chicken and chickpeas with bulgur wheat (makes 2, freeze 1)
- ★ smoky paprika popcorn

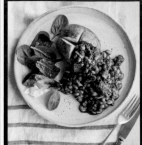
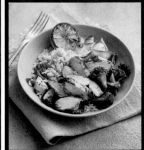
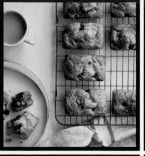
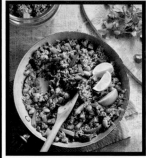
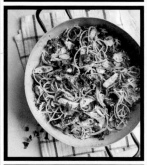
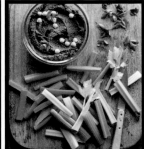
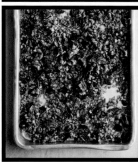
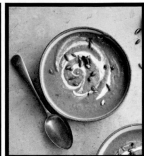
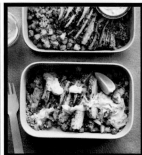
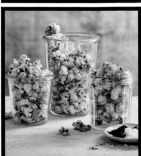
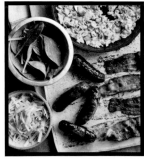
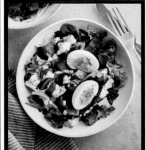

Menu for week 1

BREAKFAST	LUNCH	DINNER	SNACK
Sunday (meal prep day)			
Banana and blueberry miniature loaf *(eat 1 and freeze 9)* (216 cals)	Jacket potato with pork and BBQ beans (496 cals)	Butter bean and vegetable biryani *(make double batch and freeze half)* (455 cals)	Beetroot hummus (155 cals)
Monday			
Homemade granola (325 cals)	Turmeric chicken with rice and greens (453 cals)	Leftover jacket potato with pork and BBQ beans (496 cals)	Protein ball *(freeze 8)* (158 cals)
Tuesday			
Homemade granola (325 cals)	Leftover turmeric chicken with rice and greens (453 cals)	Leftover butter bean and vegetable biryani (455 cals)	Leftover beetroot hummus (155 cals)
Wednesday (second meal prep day)			
Banana and blueberry miniature loaf *(from freezer)* (216 cals)	Garlic chicken and kale spaghetti (492 cals)	Super green soup *(make double batch and freeze half)* (188 cals)	Leftover protein ball (158 cals)
Thursday			
Full English breakfast wrap *(eat 1 and freeze 3)* (400 cals)	Leftover garlic chicken and kale spaghetti (492 cals)	Fridge forage vegetable and lentil bowls (406 cals)	Beetroot hummus *(from freezer)* (155 cals)
Friday			
Banana and blueberry miniature loaf *(from freezer)* (216 cals)	Leftover super green soup (188 cals)	Leftover fridge forage vegetable and lentil bowls (406 cals)	Smoky paprika popcorn (165 cals)
Saturday			
Full English breakfast wrap *(from freezer)* (400 cals)	Harissa chicken and chickpeas with bulgur wheat (488 cals)	Butter bean and vegetable biryani *(from freezer)* (455 cals)	Leftover smoky paprika popcorn (165 cals)

WEEK 2

To make on the first meal prep day:
- ★ Charlotte's lasagne (double quantity –
  freeze 6 of the 8 portions)
- ★ Korean-style beef noodles
- ★ red pepper and tomato soup (double quantity
  – freeze all 4 portions for defrosting later on)
- ★ chocolate-covered roasted chickpeas
  (makes 5 portions, freeze 3) and malt
  bread (makes 10 slices, freeze 9)

To make on the second meal prep day:
- ★ fully loaded dirty fries
- ★ chorizo and feta salad with red pepper dressing
- ★ goat's cheese and caramelized onion frittata
  (freeze 2 of the 4 portions)

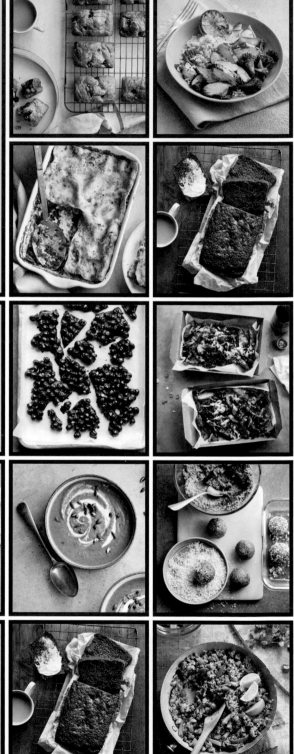

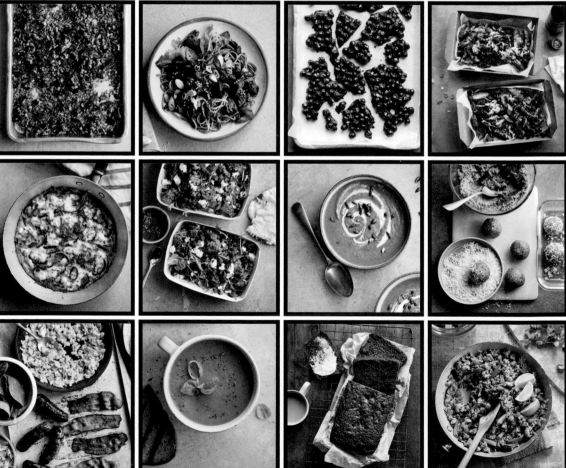

Menu for week 2

BREAKFAST	LUNCH	DINNER	SNACK
Sunday (meal prep day)			
Banana and blueberry miniature loaf *(from freezer)* (216 cals)	Harissa chicken and chickpeas with bulgur wheat *(from freezer)* (488 cals)	Charlotte's lasagne *(make double and freeze 6 portions)* (478 cals)	Malt bread *(eat 1 slice and freeze the rest)* (246 cals)
Monday			
Homemade granola (325 cals)	Korean-style beef noodles (398 cals)	Leftover Charlotte's lasagne (478 cals)	Chocolate-covered roasted chickpeas *(freeze 3 portions)* (168 cals)
Tuesday			
Banana and blueberry miniature loaf *(from freezer)* (216 cals)	Super green soup *(from freezer)* (188 cals)	Leftover Korean-style beef noodles (398 cals)	Malt bread *(from freezer)* (246 cals)
Wednesday (second meal prep day)			
Homemade granola (325 cals)	Charlotte's lasagne *(from freezer)* (478 cals)	Fully loaded dirty fries (482 cals)	Leftover chocolate-covered roasted chickpeas (168 cals)
Thursday			
Goat's cheese and caramelized onion frittata (248 cals)	Chorizo and feta salad with red pepper dressing (460 cals)	Super green soup *(from freezer)* (188 cals)	Protein ball *(from freezer)* (158 cals)
Friday			
Full English breakfast wrap *(from freezer)* (400 cals)	Red pepper and tomato soup *(from freezer)* (207 cals)	Leftover fully loaded dirty fries (482 cals)	Malt bread *(from freezer)* (246 cals)
Saturday			
Leftover goat's cheese and caramelized onion frittata (248 cals)	Leftover chorizo and feta salad with red pepper dressing (460 cals)	Butter bean and vegetable biryani *(from freezer)* (455 cals)	Protein ball *(from freezer)* (158 cals)

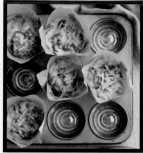

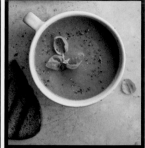

WEEK 3

To make on the first meal prep day:
★ tuna, cheese and egg muffins
  (makes 8, freeze 7)
★ cottage pie (double quantity – freeze
  2 of the 4 portions)
★ roast chicken and vegetable traybake
★ raspberry pots and sweet potato brownies
  (makes 9, freeze 8)

To make on the second meal prep day:
★ one-pot chorizo and chickpea stew
★ sausage and vegetable traybake

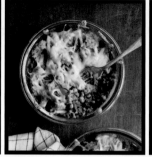

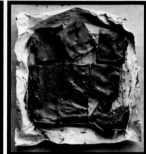

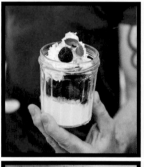

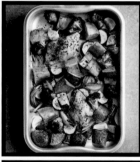

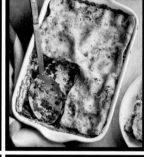

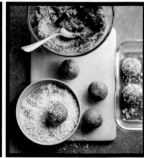

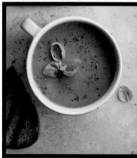

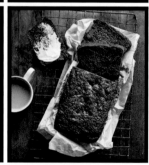

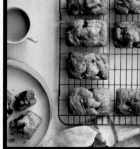

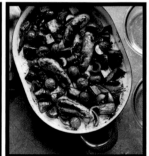

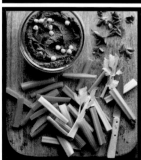

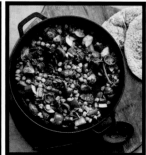

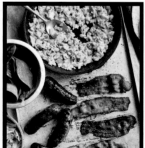

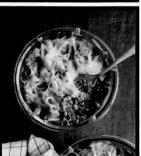

Menu for week 3

BREAKFAST	LUNCH	DINNER	SNACK
Sunday (meal prep day)			
Tuna, cheese and egg muffins *(eat 1 and freeze the rest)* (122 cals)	Roasted red pepper and tomato soup *(from freezer)* (207 cals)	Comforting cottage pie *(make double batch and freeze half)* (467 cals)	Sweet potato brownie *(eat 1 and freeze the rest)* (224 cals)
Monday			
Raspberry pot (215 cals)	Roast chicken and vegetable traybake (460 cals)	Charlotte's lasagne *(from freezer)* (478 cals)	Protein ball *(from freezer)* (158 cals)
Tuesday			
Leftover raspberry pot (215 cals)	Roasted red pepper and tomato soup *(from freezer)* (207 cals)	Leftover comforting cottage pie (467 cals)	Malt bread *(from freezer)* (246 cals)
Wednesday (second meal prep day)			
Tuna, cheese and egg muffin *(from freezer)* (122 cals)	Leftover roast chicken and vegetable traybake (460 cals)	One-pot chorizo and chickpea stew (479 cals)	Sweet potato brownie *(from freezer)* (224 cals)
Thursday			
Banana and blueberry miniature loaf *(from freezer)* (216 cals)	Leftover one-pot chorizo and chickpea stew (479 cals)	Sausage and vegetable traybake (494 cals)	Beetroot hummus *(from freezer)* (155 cals)
Friday			
Tuna, cheese and egg muffin *(from freezer)* (122 cals)	Comforting cottage pie *(from freezer)* (467 cals)	Leftover sausage and vegetable traybake (494 cals)	Banana and blueberry mini loaf *(from freezer)* (216 cals)
Saturday			
Full English breakfast wrap *(from freezer)* (400 cals)	Roasted red pepper and tomato soup *(from freezer)* (207 cals)	Charlotte's lasagne *(from freezer)* (478 cals)	Sweet potato brownie *(from freezer)* (224 cals)

A WELL-STOCKED FREEZER

Your freezer will be stocked up with the following, so you'll have meals already cooked and ready to go over the upcoming weeks:

Breakfast:

1. banana and blueberry miniature loaves (**3 portions**)
2. homemade granola (**6 portions**)
3. goat's cheese and caramelized onion frittata (**2 portions**)
4. tuna, cheese and egg muffins (**5 portions**)

Mains:

5. Charlotte's lasagne (**3 portions**)
6. cottage pie (**1 portion**)

Snacks:

7. beetroot hummus (**1 portion**)
8. protein balls (**5 portions**)
9. malt bread (**6 slices**)
10. chocolate-covered chickpeas (**3 portions**)
11. sweet potato brownies (**6 portions**)

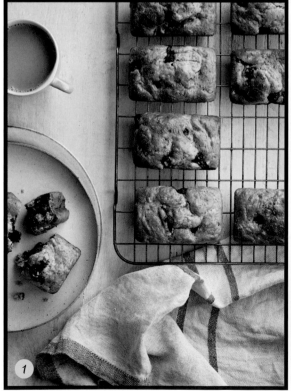

1

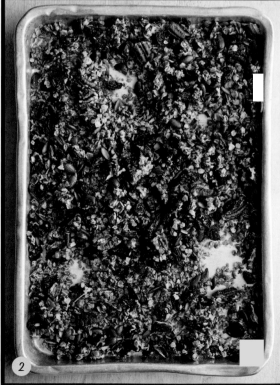

2

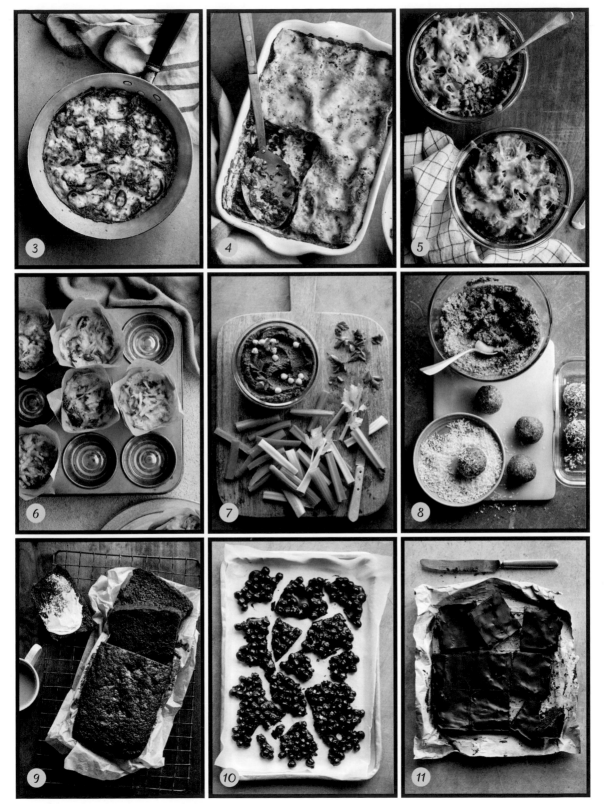

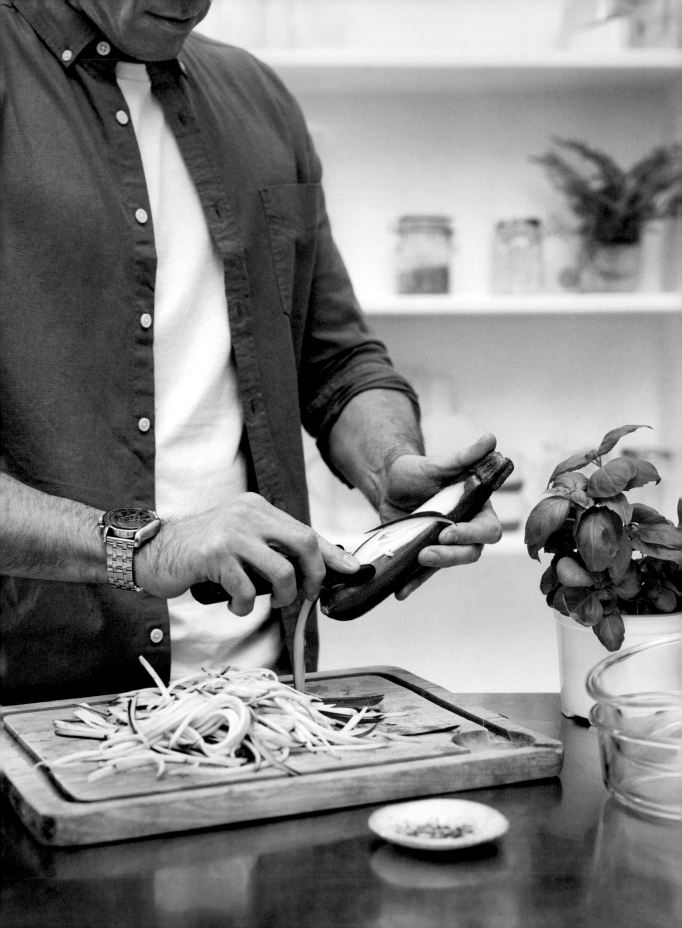

Shopping List: Week 1

FRUIT, VEGETABLES AND FRESH HERBS

- [ ] 200g bananas
- [ ] 300g blueberries
- [ ] 4 lemons
- [ ] 1 lime
- [ ] 4 onions
- [ ] 1 beetroot (or 1 packet of cooked beetroot)
- [ ] 4 carrots
- [ ] 2 jacket potatoes
- [ ] 13 cloves of garlic
- [ ] 5 sticks of celery
- [ ] 1/2 a cucumber
- [ ] 1 bag of mixed salad leaves
- [ ] 200g packet of mixed vegetables
- [ ] 100g mushrooms (optional)
- [ ] 2 red peppers
- [ ] 200g green beans
- [ ] 60g kale
- [ ] 120g spinach
- [ ] 200g tenderstem broccoli
- [ ] 200g winter greens
- [ ] 1 yellow courgette
- [ ] a large bunch of coriander
- [ ] a small handful of flat-leaf parsley (optional: another handful)
- [ ] fresh ginger

MEAT AND FISH

- [ ] 5 rashers of bacon
- [ ] 4 low-fat sausages
- [ ] 1 pork medallion
- [ ] 6 chicken breasts

DAIRY AND EGGS

- [ ] 30g butter
- [ ] 120g low-fat Cheddar cheese
- [ ] 6–8 tbsp semi-skimmed milk
- [ ] 20g Parmesan cheese
- [ ] 195g natural yoghurt
- [ ] 100g fat-free yoghurt
- [ ] 2 tbsp fat-free Greek yoghurt
- [ ] 9 eggs

TINNED GOODS

- [ ] 2 x 400g tins of butter beans
- [ ] 2 x 400g tins of chickpeas
- [ ] 1 x 400g tin of haricot beans
- [ ] 1 x 400g tin of chopped tomatoes

FROZEN

- [ ] 400g frozen broccoli florets
- [ ] 100g frozen peas

GENERAL

- [ ] 50g almonds
- [ ] 30g nut butter
- [ ] 110g pecan nuts
- [ ] 40g pumpkin seeds
- [ ] 85g peanut butter
- [ ] 40g popcorn
- [ ] 75g pitted dates
- [ ] 100g raisins
- [ ] 50g bulgur wheat
- [ ] 120g Puy lentils
- [ ] 150g passata
- [ ] 4 mini tortilla wraps
- [ ] 20g vanilla protein powder
- [ ] 120g wholegrain spaghetti

STORE CUPBOARD

- [ ] baking powder
- [ ] bicarbonate of soda
- [ ] brown sugar (or coconut sugar)
- [ ] honey
- [ ] 380g oats
- [ ] vanilla extract
- [ ] self-raising flour
- [ ] wholemeal flour
- [ ] sunflower seeds
- [ ] 1 small jar of minced garlic
- [ ] 1 small jar of minced ginger
- [ ] allspice
- [ ] cayenne pepper
- [ ] chilli powder
- [ ] garam masala
- [ ] garlic powder
- [ ] garlic salt
- [ ] ground cinnamon
- [ ] ground coriander
- [ ] ground cumin
- [ ] ground nutmeg
- [ ] ground turmeric
- [ ] harissa seasoning
- [ ] mustard powder
- [ ] onion granules
- [ ] onion salt
- [ ] paprika (or dried mixed herbs)
- [ ] smoked paprika
- [ ] 320g basmati rice
- [ ] tomato purée
- [ ] vegetable stock cubes
- [ ] light soy sauce
- [ ] low-cal spray oil
- [ ] olive oil
- [ ] salt and pepper
- [ ] sea salt

Shopping List: Week 2

FRUIT, VEGETABLES AND FRESH HERBS

- [ ] 1 lime (optional)
- [ ] 2 onions
- [ ] 400g shallot onions
- [ ] 650g white potatoes
- [ ] 1 red onion
- [ ] 12 cloves of garlic
- [ ] 1 green pepper
- [ ] 5 red peppers
- [ ] 1 red chilli (optional)
- [ ] 3 spring onions (optional)
- [ ] 200g sweet pointed pepper
- [ ] sweety drop peppers (optional)
- [ ] 600g baby plum tomatoes
- [ ] 40g rocket
- [ ] 1 bag of mixed salad (optional: an extra bag)
- [ ] 140g spring greens
- [ ] 50g kale
- [ ] 2 large bunches of basil
- [ ] a few sprigs of fresh parsley

MEAT AND FISH

- [ ] 60g chorizo
- [ ] 950g 5% fat lean beef mince
- [ ] 225g lean rump steak

DAIRY AND EGGS

- [ ] 50g unsalted butter
- [ ] 40g low-fat Cheddar cheese
- [ ] 60g feta cheese
- [ ] 60g goat's cheese
- [ ] 60g Parmesan cheese
- [ ] 400g fresh egg lasagne sheets
- [ ] 780ml semi-skimmed milk
- [ ] single cream
- [ ] 9 eggs

TINNED GOODS

- [ ] 1 x 400g tin of chickpeas

GENERAL

- [ ] 60g black treacle
- [ ] 60g malt extract
- [ ] 100g caster sugar (optional)
- [ ] 1 tsp cornflour
- [ ] 100g dark chocolate
- [ ] 90g golden syrup
- [ ] 170g sultanas or raisins
- [ ] 1/2 tsp hot chilli sauce
- [ ] 800g passata
- [ ] 20ml apple cider vinegar
- [ ] balsamic glaze (optional)
- [ ] 1 tsp rice vinegar
- [ ] sriracha (optional)
- [ ] 100g wholegrain noodles
- [ ] wholemeal pitta bread (optional)

STORE CUPBOARD

- [ ] honey*
- [ ] light brown sugar
- [ ] plain flour
- [ ] self-raising flour*
- [ ] sweetener
- [ ] allspice*
- [ ] bay leaves
- [ ] chilli flakes
- [ ] Chinese five-spice powder
- [ ] dried oregano
- [ ] onion salt*
- [ ] sesame seeds (optional)
- [ ] low-cal spray oil*
- [ ] olive oil*
- [ ] soy sauce*
- [ ] Worcestershire sauce
- [ ] vegetable oil
- [ ] salt and pepper*
- [ ] ground black pepper
- [ ] sea salt*
- [ ] white pepper
- [ ] chicken or vegetable* stock cubes

All the ingredients with an asterisk (*) next to them may have been bought in the week before.

Shopping List: Week 3

FRUIT, VEGETABLES AND FRESH HERBS

- [ ] 1 lemon
- [ ] 1 lime
- [ ] 100g raspberries
- [ ] 2 carrots
- [ ] 2 onions
- [ ] 2 red onions
- [ ] 10 cloves of garlic
- [ ] 800g sweet potatoes
- [ ] 2 sticks of celery
- [ ] 400g cherry tomatoes
- [ ] 50g spring onions
- [ ] 2 red peppers
- [ ] 100g spinach
- [ ] 1 aubergine
- [ ] 200g broccoli
- [ ] 2 courgettes
- [ ] a small handful of flat-leaf parsley
- [ ] a few sprigs of mint
- [ ] a small handful of thyme

MEAT AND FISH

- [ ] 500g 5% fat lean beef mince
- [ ] 2 chicken thigh fillets
- [ ] 50g chorizo sausage
- [ ] 4 sausages

DAIRY AND EGGS

- [ ] 90g low-fat Cheddar cheese
- [ ] 30g Parmesan cheese
- [ ] 40ml semi-skimmed milk
- [ ] 300g low-fat Greek yoghurt
- [ ] low-fat squirty cream (optional)
- [ ] 9 eggs

TINNED GOODS

- [ ] 1 x 400g tin of chickpeas
- [ ] 1 x 200g tin of sweetcorn
- [ ] 2 x 400g tins of plum tomatoes
- [ ] 1 x 145g tin of tuna

FROZEN

- [ ] 100g frozen peas

GENERAL

- [ ] 100g dark chocolate
- [ ] 2 digestive biscuits
- [ ] 125g nut butter
- [ ] 30g unsweetened cocoa powder
- [ ] 2 wholegrain pitta breads (optional)

STORE CUPBOARD

- [ ] baking powder
- [ ] brown sugar*
- [ ] flaxseeds
- [ ] honey*
- [ ] sweetener*
- [ ] balsamic vinegar
- [ ] vanilla extract*
- [ ] bay leaf*
- [ ] ground coriander*
- [ ] ground cumin*
- [ ] smoked paprika*
- [ ] low-cal spray oil*
- [ ] olive oil*
- [ ] Worcestershire sauce*
- [ ] salt and pepper*
- [ ] beef stock cube
- [ ] vegetable stock cube*
- [ ] tomato purée*

All the ingredients with an asterisk (*) next to them may have been bought in the weeks before.

CREATE YOUR OWN 21-DAY PLAN

The beauty of meal prep is that you can mix and match the meals as you see fit so that it works around your day-to-day life. You might not want to follow my set 21-day plan, so I've included three blank grids on the next few pages so that you can create your own. You might want to be meat-free on a certain number of days a week or you might be like me and sometimes want to have the breakfast wrap for dinner and the sweet potato brownies for breakfast – whatever takes your fancy! Have fun and experiment with different meal prep plans.

Make sure to include the calorie breakdown from the recipes so that you'll know how many calories you're consuming a day, and always check what you have left in your fridge so you can create recipes around your leftovers. I'd love to see the meal prep plans you come up with! Feel free to share them with me online using the hashtag #TMPKplan.

'Have fun and experiment with different meal prep plans…whatever takes your fancy!'

MENU FOR WEEK 1

BREAKFAST	LUNCH	DINNER	SNACK
Sunday			
Monday			
Tuesday			
Wednesday			
Thursday			
Friday			
Saturday			

MENU FOR WEEK 2

BREAKFAST	LUNCH	DINNER	SNACK
Sunday			
Monday			
Tuesday			
Wednesday			
Thursday			
Friday			
Saturday			

MENU FOR WEEK 3

BREAKFAST	LUNCH	DINNER	SNACK
Sunday			
Monday			
Tuesday			
Wednesday			
Thursday			
Friday			
Saturday			

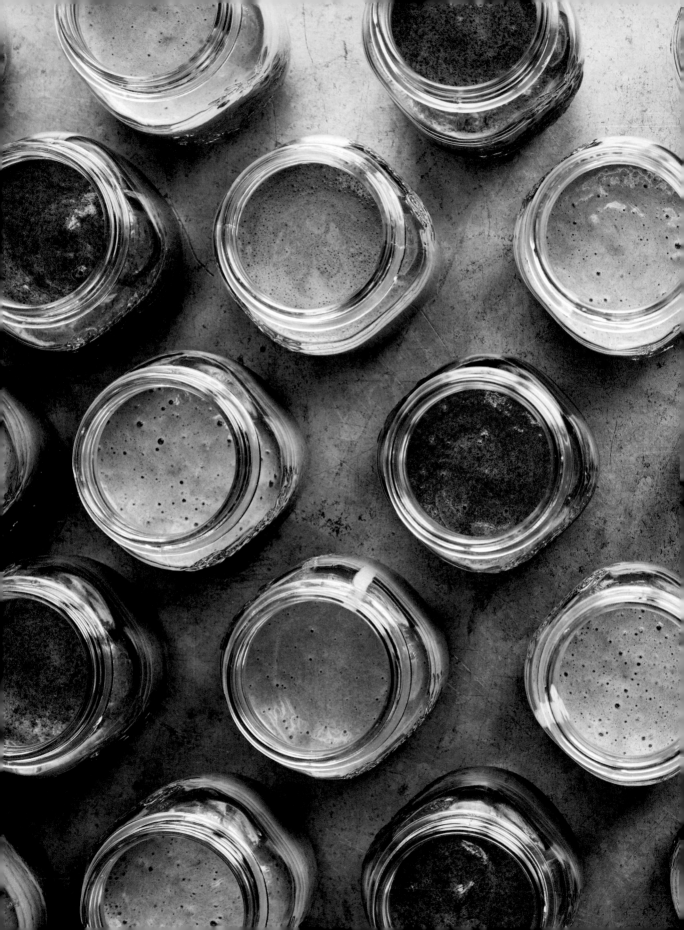

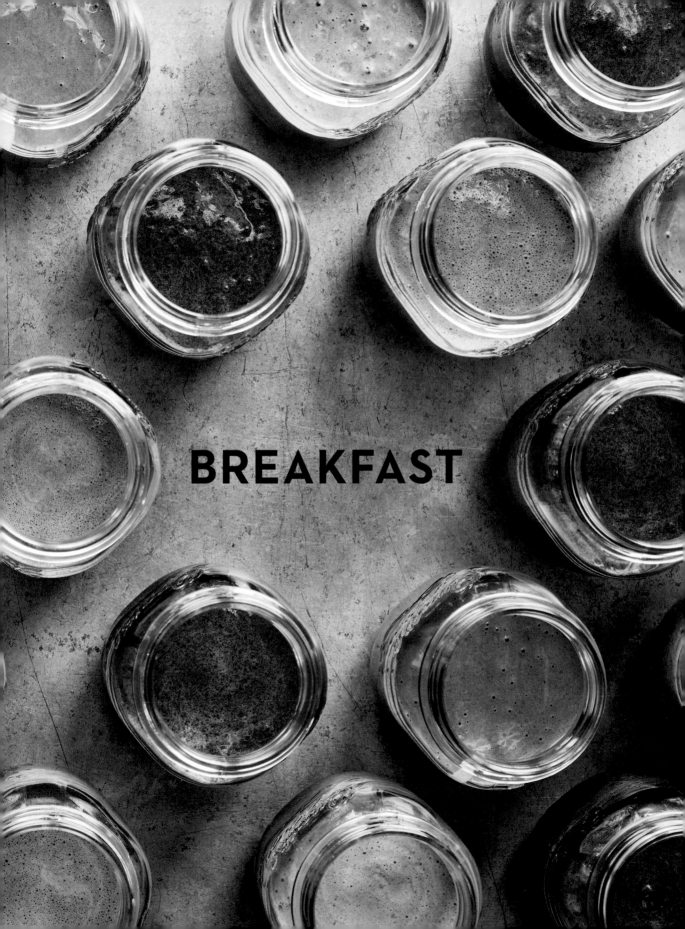

BREAKFAST

FULL ENGLISH BREAKFAST WRAP

PER SERVING | 400 CALS | 27G PROTEIN | 24G FAT | 17G CARBS

10 MINS   25 MINS   FREEZE

MAKES 4 WRAPS

4 rashers of bacon
4 low-fat sausages
4 mini tortilla wraps
120g low-fat Cheddar
   cheese
20g spinach
4 eggs
20g butter, cubed
salt and pepper

*If you're going to freeze
these wraps, don't include
the spinach as you can
add fresh spinach after
you reheat it.*

*Fast-food full English breakfast wraps are absolutely
delicious so I'm going to show you how you can make your
own guilt-free ones at home. They also freeze beautifully.
Tuck in!*

1 Cook your bacon and sausages according to the pack
instructions – I find it easiest just to pop them in the oven.

2 Lay out four mini tortillas and add 30g of cheese per wrap,
then add a layer of spinach and a slice of bacon per tortilla.
Cut each cooked sausage in half and add to the wrap.

3 Lastly, put the four eggs and butter into a bowl, mix and
season. Heat a frying pan over a medium heat, then add the
egg mixture, stirring continuously until cooked. Divide
the egg evenly between the four tortilla wraps.

4 Fold baking paper around each wrap, so you can eat
them easily after you reheat them, and store in an airtight
container in the fridge for up to 3 days. They will keep
for up to 3 months in the freezer.

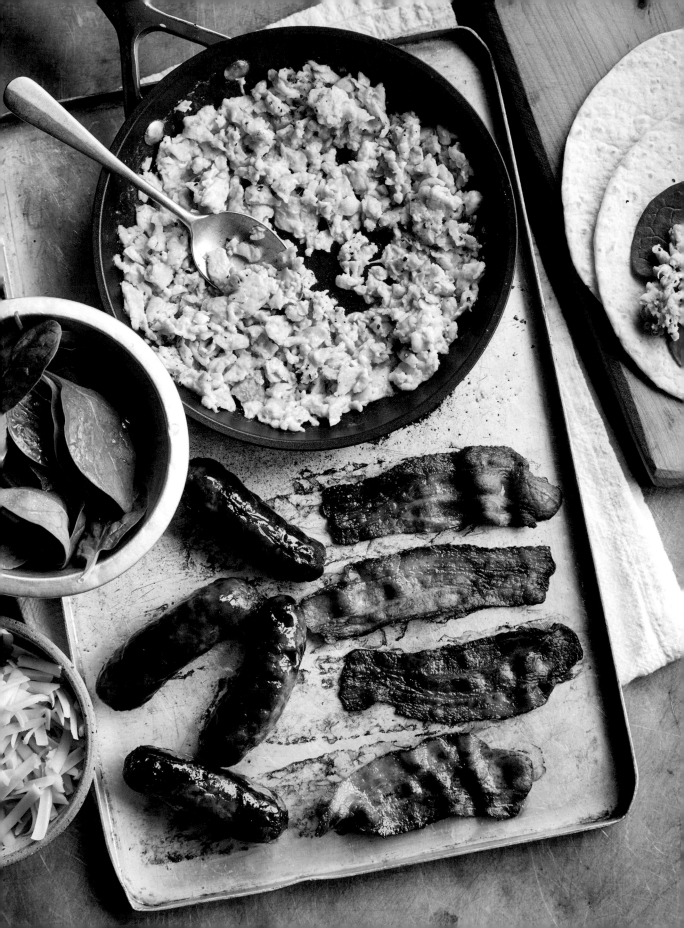

BREAKFAST PROTEIN BARS

PER SERVING | **249** CALS | **11G** PROTEIN | **12G** FAT | **24G** CARBS

10 MINS | **FREEZE**

MAKES 10 BARS

30g honey
130g smooth nut butter
100ml milk
a pinch of salt
50g vanilla whey protein
    powder (or your
    preferred flavour)
200g rolled porridge oats
100g dark chocolate
    (at least 70% cocoa)

Shop-bought protein bars are so expensive – let me show you how you can make your own for a fraction of the price! These are a firm favourite in our house and you can bung them into the freezer to use at a later date. They make a fun healthy snack for the kids, too.

1 Put the honey, nut butter, milk and salt into a saucepan over a low heat and stir to combine. Once it's smooth and warmed through, remove from the heat and stir in the protein powder.

2 Add the porridge oats and mix thoroughly. The dough should be firm but pliable. If it's too dry, just add more milk, a little at a time, until you reach the desired consistency.

3 Line a baking tray with baking paper. Put the mixture on to the tray and use a spatula to flatten it out into one giant bar. Melt 100g of your favourite chocolate (you can do this in short bursts in the microwave or in a heatproof bowl over a saucepan of boiling water) and spread a layer over the top of the mixture so it's all covered.

4 Place in the freezer for a couple of hours (I like mine firm and it does speed up the process). However, if you prefer yours a little more on the gooey side, just pop the tray straight into the fridge for a couple of hours. Once set, cut into 10 bars. They will keep for up to 5 days in the fridge in an airtight container or in the freezer for up to 3 months.

CLASSIC CHEESE SCONES

PER SERVING | **122** CALS | **5G** PROTEIN | **4G** FAT | **16G** CARBS

15 MINS   20 MINS   FREEZE

MAKES 10 SCONES

200g self-raising flour
1 tsp salt
1 tsp mustard powder
30g low-fat margarine
75g low-fat Cheddar
   cheese, grated
1 large egg
60ml skimmed milk, plus
   a little extra to glaze
low-cal spray oil

Cheese scones are a true traditional classic and these light and fluffy ones are perfect spread with low-fat margarine for a tasty breakfast.

1 Preheat the oven to 200°C. Mix the self-raising flour, salt and mustard powder together in a bowl. Then add the low-fat margarine, rubbing it into the flour to form a light breadcrumb texture. Stir in 55g of the low-fat Cheddar cheese.

2 In a separate bowl, whisk the egg and milk together. Slowly pour this into the dry ingredients and mix until you have a fairly firm dough.

3 Roll the dough out on a lightly floured surface to a thickness of approximately 2cm. Cut out the scones using an 8cm cutter (or an upturned glass if you don't have a cutter).

4 Line a baking tray with baking paper and spray with low-cal oil. Place the scones on it and brush them with a little milk. Top them with the remaining 20g of cheese.

5 Bake in the oven for 15–20 minutes until golden brown. The scones will keep in a sealed container for up to 3 days or in the freezer for up to 3 months.

POPPY-SEED PANCAKES

PER SERVING | **273** CALS | **29G** PROTEIN | **8G** FAT | **20G** CARBS

5 MINS   5 MINS   FREEZE

SERVES 2

50g porridge oats
50g vanilla whey protein
   powder (or your
   preferred flavour)
1 egg
1/4 tsp baking powder
100ml milk
1 tsp poppy seeds
low-cal spray oil

To serve:
fruit of your choice
honey, to drizzle

Another easy breakfast meal that you can either keep in the fridge or freeze. Top with seasonal fruit, which you can buy at bargain prices from the market.

1 Blend the porridge oats to a fine powder in a food processor. Pour into a bowl along with the protein powder, egg, baking powder, milk and poppy seeds and stir to combine until smooth.

2 Heat a small frying pan over a medium heat. Spritz the pan with some low-cal oil and spoon in 2 tablespoons of the batter. Fry for 1–2 minutes per side until the pancake is golden brown.

3 The pancakes will keep in the fridge for up to 3 days or in the freezer for up to 3 months. Serve topped with fresh fruit and drizzled with honey (remember to count the extra calories).

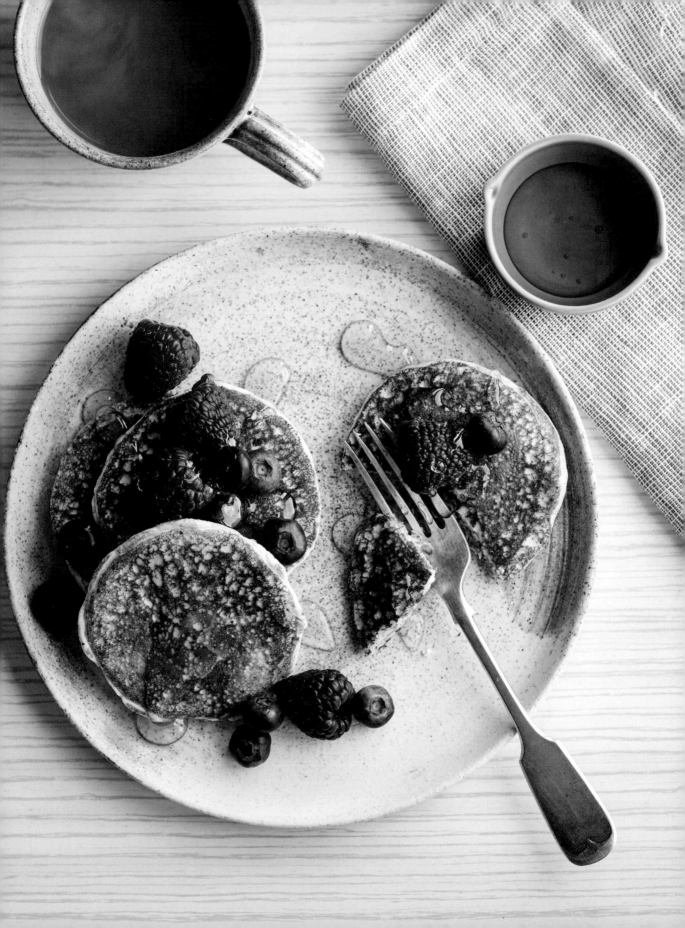

HOMEMADE GRANOLA

PER SERVING | **325** CALS | **6G** PROTEIN | **19G** FAT | **32G** CARBS

5 MINS   30 MINS   FREEZE

SERVES 10

280g porridge oats
100g raisins
40g pumpkin seeds
80g pecan nuts, chopped
20g brown sugar
50g honey
90g olive oil
1 tsp sea salt
1/2 tsp ground cinnamon

The benefit of making your own granola is that you can skip the refined sugar and other bad things often found in supermarket versions. And this homemade one is not only healthier but also cheaper. Feel free to experiment with different nuts, seeds and dried fruits – the combinations are endless!

1 Preheat the oven to 180°C. Line a baking tray with baking paper (top tip: spray the baking tray with oil before lining it as it will help the baking paper stick down).

2 Mix all the ingredients together thoroughly to combine, making sure that everything is coated in the oil. Tip the mixture on to the baking tray and even it out with a spatula. Place in the oven for 30 minutes, turning the granola once halfway through, until golden brown.

3 The granola can be kept in an airtight container for up to 6 months or in the freezer for 3 months. Serve with fresh cold skimmed milk or enjoy as part of a snack.

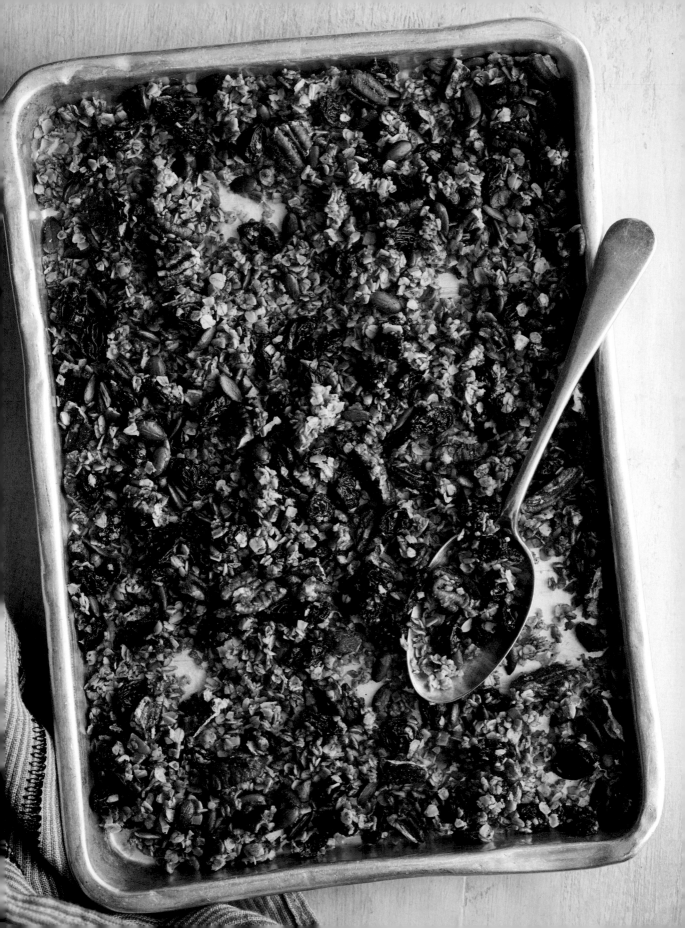

BLACK FOREST OVERNIGHT OATS

PER SERVING | **449** CALS | **26G** PROTEIN | **13G** FAT | **53G** CARBS

prep

10 MINS

SERVES 2

80g rolled oats
15g cocoa powder
20g chia seeds
20g agave syrup or honey
30g chocolate whey
    protein powder
1/2 tsp vanilla extract
1/4 tsp ground cinnamon
260ml semi-skimmed milk
80g frozen cherries
1 tbsp chocolate chips
    or chunks
optional: 10g goji berries

Who doesn't like the flavour of cherries mixed with chocolate? I absolutely love making things that feel like treats but are full of nutrients, and this is one of those recipes!

1 Place 40g of the oats in each of two Mason jars (about 600ml in capacity) or two airtight containers. Divide the cocoa powder, chia seeds, agave syrup or honey, chocolate whey protein powder, vanilla extract and cinnamon equally between the portions and mix.

2 Add half the milk to each container, followed by the frozen cherries, and mix again. Seal and leave overnight in the fridge.

3 These oats will keep in the fridge for up to 3 days. To serve, sprinkle over the chocolate chips, and if you want to add a bit of a texture, some goji berries.

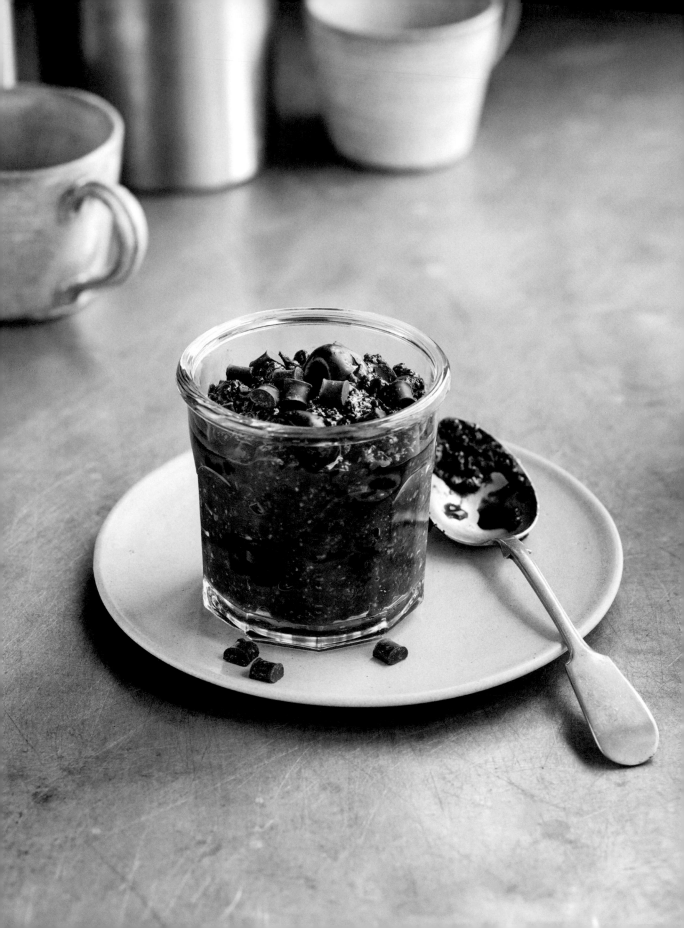

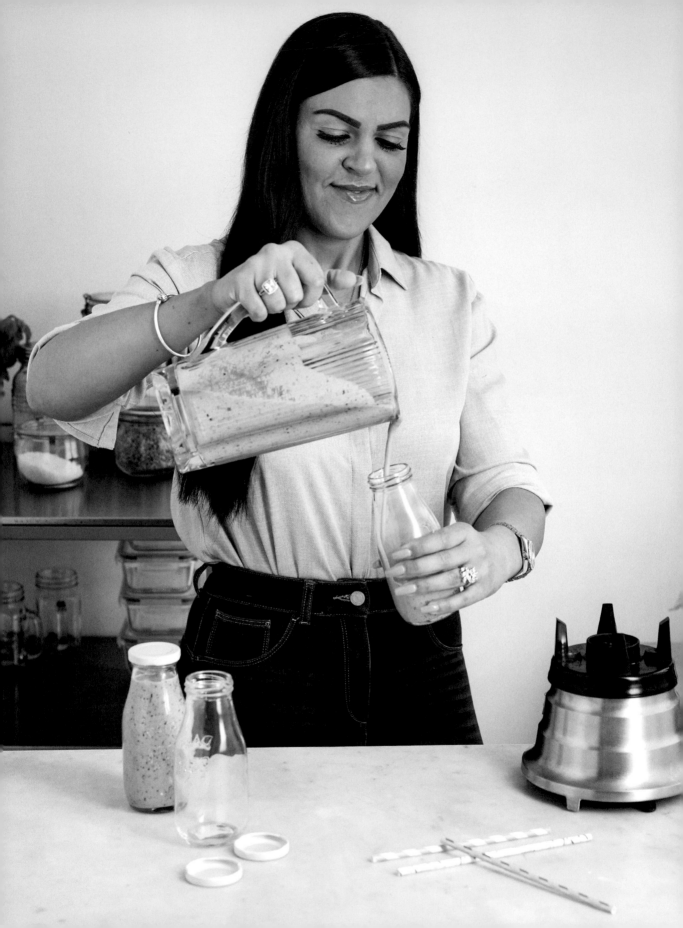

Smoothies are fantastic for using up any spare fruit and
a great way to consume a lot of nutrients in one sitting.

PROTEIN-PACKED SUPERFOOD SHAKE

PER SERVING | **443** CALS | **32G** PROTEIN | **11G** FAT | **49G** CARBS

5 MINS · FREEZE

SERVES 2

2 frozen bananas
100g frozen blueberries
100g frozen strawberries
100g frozen raspberries
100g frozen cherries
60g whey protein
40g linseed or flaxseed
30g honey

To serve:
chia seeds
linseed or flaxseed

*I'm a huge advocate of nutritional benefits so this smoothie
ticks a lot of boxes. The brightly coloured berries and cherries
are rich in anthocyanins (plant pigments), which help promote
heart health, reduce inflammation and lower blood pressure.
They are also packed with vitamin C, important for good
immunity and healthy blood vessels. Flaxseeds are rich
in omega-3s, which support brain health, protect against
heart disease and may help treat depression. Drink up!*

1 Blend all the ingredients together in a food processor with
500ml water. Once everything is blended you can adjust the
thickness to your desired consistency using water or crushed
ice. This smoothie will keep in the fridge for 3 days or in the
freezer for up to 3 months. Serve topped with chia seeds
and extra flaxseed or linseed.

DOUBLE-CHOCOLATE MINT SMOOTHIE

PER SERVING | **393** CALS | **29G** PROTEIN | **24G** FAT | **13G** CARBS

prep

5 MINS

FREEZE

SERVES 2

50g chocolate
　protein powder
40g hazelnuts
30g cocoa powder
2 tbsp chocolate chips
400ml almond milk
8 fresh mint leaves
a handful of ice cubes

To serve:
chocolate chips

If you want a really chocolatey smoothie, try using chocolate almond milk for an extra kick!

It's no secret that mint is chocolate's best friend and they make the perfect combination. With hazelnuts and fresh mint, this tastes more like a dessert than a smoothie. You won't be disappointed.

1 Blend all the ingredients together in a food processor. Once everything is blended you can adjust the thickness to your desired consistency using water or extra almond milk. Just remember to add the extra calories if using extra almond milk. This smoothie will keep in the fridge for 3 days or in the freezer for up to 3 months. Serve topped with extra chocolate chips.

POMEGRANATE SMOOTHIE

PER SERVING | **323** CALS | **5G** PROTEIN | **13G** FAT | **41G** CARBS

5 MINS FREEZE

SERVES 2

250g fresh pomegranate
  seeds
200g frozen raspberries
1 banana, roughly chopped
10 ice cubes
juice of 1 lemon
300ml light coconut milk

To serve:
chia seeds
crushed almonds
shavings of white chocolate

Pomegranates contain high levels of antioxidants, which are known to protect cells from damage and reduce inflammation. They're also high in vitamin C, potassium and fibre. Did you know that most of the fibre that comes from pomegranates is found in the seeds? And the best bit is that they taste great!

1 Blend all the ingredients together in a food processor with 150–200ml water. Once everything is blended you can adjust the thickness to your desired consistency using water or extra coconut milk. Just remember to add the extra calories if using extra coconut milk. This smoothie will keep in the fridge for 3 days or in the freezer for up to 3 months. Serve topped with chia seeds, crushed almonds and shavings of white chocolate.

BANANA & BLUEBERRY MINIATURE LOAVES

PER SERVING (1 MINI LOAF OR 1 SLICE) | **216** CALS | **8G** PROTEIN | **6G** FAT | **30G** CARBS

10 MINS   30 MINS MINI   1 HOUR 15 MINS LARGE   FREEZE

MAKES 10 MINI LOAVES OR 1 LARGE LOAF

150g wholemeal flour
100g self-raising flour
1 tsp bicarbonate of soda
1 tsp baking powder
1/2 tsp ground cinnamon
3 eggs
85g peanut butter
150g natural yoghurt
50g honey
1 tsp vanilla extract
200g bananas, mashed
300g blueberries

This recipe was first introduced to me by my friend Frank. I'd often visit Frank as a youngster and if I was lucky enough, I'd arrive just in time to smell these being taken out of the oven. Being from a different era, Frank incorporates baking into his routine pretty much every day and this recipe is not to be missed.

1 Preheat the oven to 170°C and grease a mini-loaf tin or large loaf tin. Combine the flours, bicarbonate of soda, baking powder and cinnamon in a bowl. In another bowl, mix the eggs, peanut butter, yoghurt, honey, vanilla extract and mashed bananas together thoroughly. Mix the wet and dry mixtures together, then stir through the blueberries.

2 If you're making one big loaf, pour the mixture into the greased loaf tin and bake for 1–1¼ hours in the middle of the oven. If you're making mini loaves, divide the mixture evenly between the holes (I use an ice-cream scoop for this!) and bake in the middle of the oven for 25–30 minutes.

3 To test that a loaf is cooked through, poke in a skewer – if it comes out clean, the loaf is ready. Remove from the oven and leave to cool for 5 minutes in the tin before tipping the loaves out. Leave to cool on a wire rack. If you made a large loaf, slice it into 10 portions. The mini loaves/slices will keep in an airtight container for 3 days or in the freezer for up to 3 months.

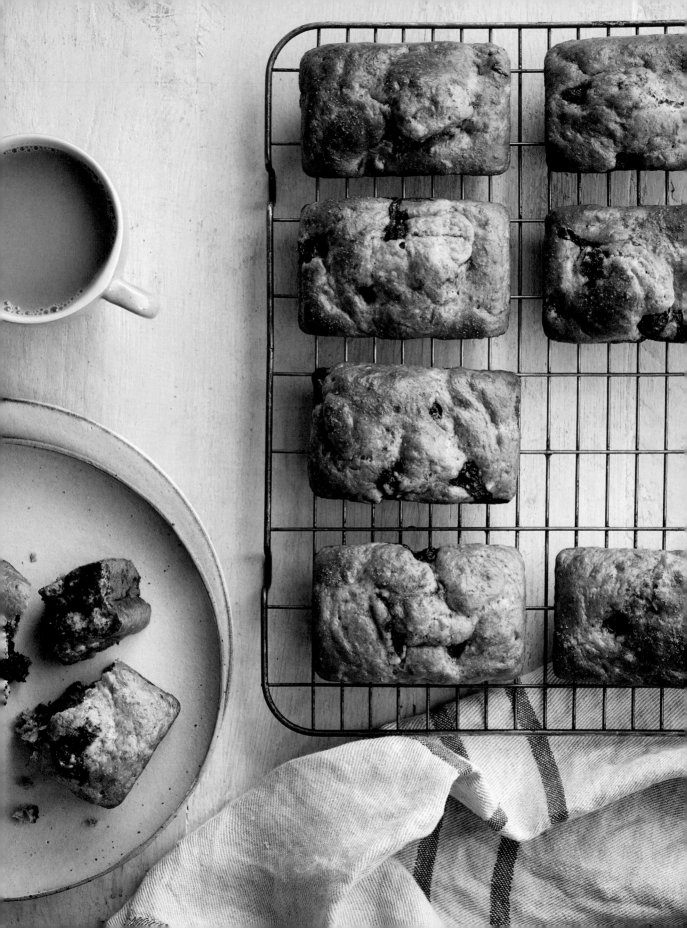

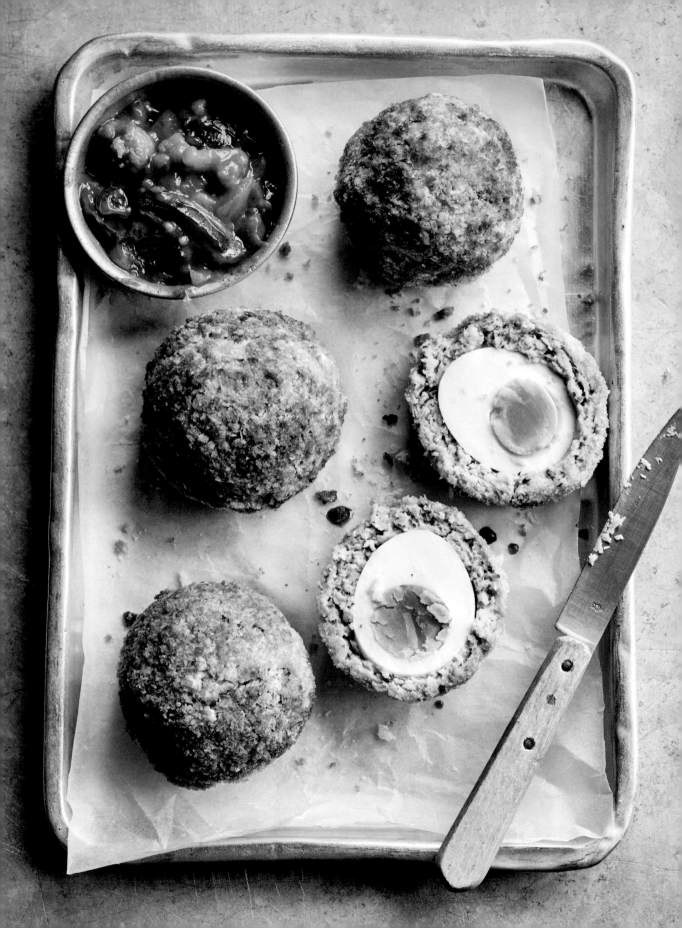

BAKED SCOTCH EGGS

PER SERVING | **289** CALS | **22G** PROTEIN | **12G** FAT | **22G** CARBS

prep **cook** **FREEZE**
20 MINS 35 MINS

MAKES 4 SCOTCH EGGS

6 eggs
300g low-fat sausages
a small handful of fresh
    parsley, finely chopped
1/4 tsp mustard powder
1/4 tsp ground marjoram
10g plain flour
75g panko breadcrumbs
low-cal spray oil
salt and pepper

These lovely Scotch eggs are great as a breakfast on the go or to eat at your desk at work, or they can be an afternoon snack. Or why not add one into the kids' lunch boxes for school? What I like about these is they are baked, not fried, which is a great way to keep the calories down. Be sure to look for good-quality sausages that are lower in fat and therefore calories as well.

1 Preheat the oven to 200°C. Put four eggs into a pan, cover them with cold water and bring the water to a boil, then turn down the heat and leave to simmer for 5 minutes. Take out the eggs and put them into a bowl of cold water – leave them to cool for at least 10 minutes.

2 Meanwhile, squeeze the sausage meat from the skins into a large bowl and mix in the finely chopped parsley, mustard powder, ground marjoram and seasoning.

3 Divide the sausage meat into four even balls, then peel the boiled eggs. Place a large piece of clingfilm on the work surface, place one of the balls in the centre and cover it with another piece of clingfilm. Roll out the sausage meat until it's large enough to cover the egg.

4 Remove the top layer of clingfilm, place a boiled egg in the middle and use the clingfilm at the sides to bring the sausage meat up so it covers the egg. Use your hands to smooth it into shape. Do the same with the remaining balls and eggs.

Recipe continued overleaf

5 Put the flour into one bowl and season it, break the two remaining eggs into a second bowl and whisk, then put the breadcrumbs into a third bowl. Dip each encased egg into the flour and then into the egg mixture before rolling them in breadcrumbs. Dip them into the egg mixture again and coat once more with the breadcrumbs.

6 Spray each egg with low-cal oil and place them on a lined baking tray. Cook them in the oven for 25–30 minutes, turning them occasionally to ensure that they brown evenly.

7 Remove the Scotch eggs from the oven and leave them to cool. I like to eat them with a little bit of mustard or shop-bought piccalilli! They will keep in the fridge for up to 3 days or in the freezer for up to 3 months.

SWEET POTATO HASH

PER SERVING | **259** CALS | **9G** PROTEIN | **11G** FAT | **29G** CARBS

10 MINS   30 MINS

SERVES 2

1 tbsp olive oil
1 sweet potato, peeled
    and cut into 5cm cubes
1 red onion
1 red pepper
1 clove of garlic, peeled
1/2 a red chilli
1/4 tsp smoked paprika
1/4 tsp ground cumin
2 eggs
1 lime, cut into wedges
salt and pepper

Optional toppings:
sliced spring onions
fresh coriander leaves,
    roughly chopped

This one-pan wonder not only saves on the washing-up but is always a winner in our house thanks to its vibrant colour and punchy flavours.

1 Heat the olive oil in a medium-sized non-stick pan (which has a lid) on a low heat. Fry the sweet potato, stirring occasionally, for 10 minutes until soft.

2 Meanwhile, slice the red onion into half-moons, deseed and slice the red pepper into strips, crush the garlic and finely dice the red chilli. Then add these to the pan along with the smoked paprika and cumin. Cover the pan and cook for 5–10 minutes, stirring occasionally, until the vegetables have started to soften. Season to taste.

3 Create two wells in the pan and break an egg into each one. Cover again and cook for 6–8 minutes until the eggs are done to your liking. Divide between two airtight containers and add the lime wedges to squeeze over the top after you've reheated the meal. Top with sliced spring onions and chopped coriander if you wish. This will keep in the fridge for up to 3 days.

TUNA, CHEESE & EGG MUFFINS

PER SERVING | 122 CALS | 14G PROTEIN | 7G FAT | 1G CARBS

prep 10 MINS **cook** 20 MINS **FREEZE**

MAKES 8 MUFFINS

8 eggs
50g spring onions
100g broccoli
70g red pepper
30g Parmesan cheese, grated
1 x 145g tin of tuna, drained
low-cal spray oil
10g low-fat Cheddar cheese, grated
salt and pepper

If you don't have a muffin tin, you can use silicone muffin cases.

These little muffins pack a serious protein punch and can be enjoyed hot or cold. They're a great alternative to a sandwich if you fancy something with virtually no carbs. They're ideal to eat on the go when you're rushing out of the house as well as a perfect post-workout snack to have after a session at the gym.

1 Preheat the oven to 180°C. Crack six eggs into a large mixing jug (I find this is easier to pour). Season and whisk.

2 Finely dice the spring onions, broccoli and red pepper and add to the whisked egg, followed by the Parmesan cheese. Combine all the ingredients well, then flake in the tuna and stir one last time.

3 Spray each muffin compartment or muffin case with low-cal spray oil and smooth it round the edges with your fingers. Divide the egg mixture equally between each compartment/case. Top each muffin with the low-fat Cheddar cheese.

4 Place in the middle of the oven and bake for 18–20 minutes until cooked through and golden brown. Enjoy them right away or leave to cool on a wire rack. They will keep in the fridge for up to 3 days or can be frozen for up to 3 months.

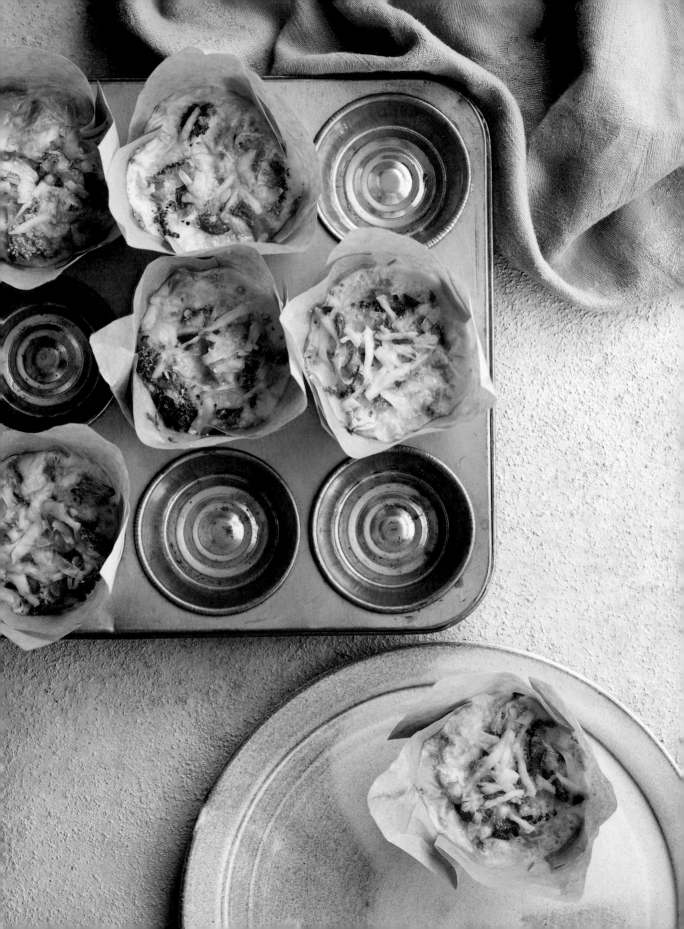

CINNAMON QUINOA FRENCH TOAST

PER SERVING | **128 CALS** | **6G PROTEIN** | **2G FAT** | **20G CARBS**

prep **5 MINS**   cook **45 MINS**   **FREEZE**

SERVES 8

200g quinoa
2 egg whites (about 75g)
1 egg
1/2 tsp ground cinnamon
20g honey, plus extra
   for drizzling
50ml semi-skimmed milk
2 tsp vanilla extract
low-cal spray oil
optional: 10g sugar
400g strawberries,
   chopped

If you're freezing this one, don't add the fruit or honey until you've reheated it so it tastes as fresh as possible.

This one will really surprise you all – it surprised me when I first made it! If you want French toast without the bread, then this is for you. I've tweaked the recipe over the years and it's now a popular breakfast choice in our house.

1 Preheat the oven to 190°C. Wash the quinoa in a sieve under cold running water to get rid of any bitterness, then put the drained quinoa into a saucepan and add 1 litre of boiling water. Simmer for 15 minutes. Drain in a sieve and squeeze out as much water as you can.

2 Put the egg whites, egg, cinnamon, honey, milk and vanilla extract into a bowl and mix thoroughly until combined. Then add the drained quinoa to the bowl and mix well.

3 Line a baking tray with baking paper and spray with low-cal spray oil to ensure it doesn't stick. Tip the quinoa mix on to the tray and smooth into the corners with the back of a spoon or a spatula to make an even layer.

4 Bake in the oven for 30 minutes until golden brown and set. Allow to cool, then sprinkle with sugar, if using, and cut into eight pieces. Drizzle with honey and either enjoy warm with chopped strawberries or allow to cool and use as meal prep. It will keep in the fridge for up to 3 days or in the freezer for up to 3 months.

SWEET OR SAVOURY SWEET POTATO WAFFLES

PER SERVING FOR SWEET VERSION | **317** CALS | **10G** PROTEIN | **3G** FAT | **58G** CARBS
PER SERVING FOR SAVOURY VERSION | **411** CALS | **13G** PROTEIN | **15G** FAT | **51G** CARBS

5 MINS **25 MINS** **FREEZE**

SERVES 2

300g sweet potatoes
60g spelt flour
1 egg
a pinch of sea salt
a pinch of black pepper
low-cal spray oil

For a sweet waffle:
10g honey
100g fresh blueberries

For a savoury waffle:
2 bacon rashers
1/2 an avocado
juice of 1/2 a lemon
1/4 tsp garlic granules
salt and pepper

You can double or triple the ingredients so you can batch-make these waffles and then freeze them for up to 3 months. Perfect for a speedy breakfast.

These sweet potato waffles are a healthy version of a Flemish classic. Will you have the sweet version or the savoury one though?

1 Peel the sweet potatoes and dice into cubes. Bring a pan of salted water to the boil and boil the sweet potatoes for 15–20 minutes until tender. Then drain and mash.

2 Mix the mashed sweet potatoes, the spelt flour, egg, sea salt and black pepper together in a bowl. Pour the mixture into a preheated, greased (I use low-cal spray oil) waffle maker and cook for about 5 minutes.

3 If you are making the sweet version, divide the honey between two small salad dressing containers. Put the waffles into two airtight containers and add the honey pots and the fruit. They will keep in the fridge for up to 3 days or in the freezer for up to 3 months.

4 If you are making the savoury version, heat a frying pan over a medium heat and fry the bacon until crispy. Allow to cool and divide between two airtight containers with the waffles. Mash the avocado in a bowl, then mix in the lemon juice, garlic granules and seasoning (it's best to do this on the day you want to eat the waffle as the avocado smash won't keep very well in the fridge). The waffles (minus the avocado) will keep in the fridge for up to 3 days or in the freezer for up to 3 months.

GOAT'S CHEESE & CARAMELIZED ONION FRITTATA

PER SERVING | **248 CALS** | **16G PROTEIN** | **16G FAT** | **10G CARBS**

prep
5 MINS

cook
30 MINS

FREEZE

SERVES 4

1 tbsp olive oil
1 large red onion, sliced
    into half moons
10g light brown sugar
20g honey
8 eggs
60g goat's cheese
a bag of mixed salad
1 lime, cut into quarters
optional: a drizzle of
    balsamic glaze
salt and pepper

To serve:
chopped chives, to garnish

tip

*If you're reheating this
after it's been frozen,
I recommend using the
oven as the microwave
might make it soggy,
though it will still taste
good. If freezing, don't
include the salad leaves.*

*This frittata is a simple and incredibly light, tasty breakfast.
The sweetness of the onions mixed with the creaminess
of the cheese makes this irresistible, so try not to eat it all
at once! Add a handful of kale or spinach to the mixture
for extra nutrients.*

1 Heat the olive oil in a large ovenproof frying pan over a
medium heat, then add the onion and sauté for 8–12 minutes
until it starts to soften. Add the brown sugar and honey to
the pan and sauté for a further 5 minutes until the onions
are nice and caramelized.

2 Preheat the grill to a medium setting. Whisk the eggs, add
the caramelized onions to the mixture and season. Return to
the pan and fry on a low heat for 3–5 minutes until the bottom
of the frittata has set.

3 Crumble the goats' cheese over the top and place under
the grill for 5 minutes until the cheese is melted and the top
is golden brown.

4 Allow to cool and slice into four quarters. Divide the salad
leaves between four airtight containers, then top each one
with a slice of frittata. Add a wedge of lime, for squeezing over,
and I like to add a drizzle of balsamic glaze for sweetness.
Garnish with chopped chives, if you like. The frittata will keep
for up to 3 days in the fridge or in the freezer (leave out the
salad) for up to 3 months. Enjoy hot or cold.

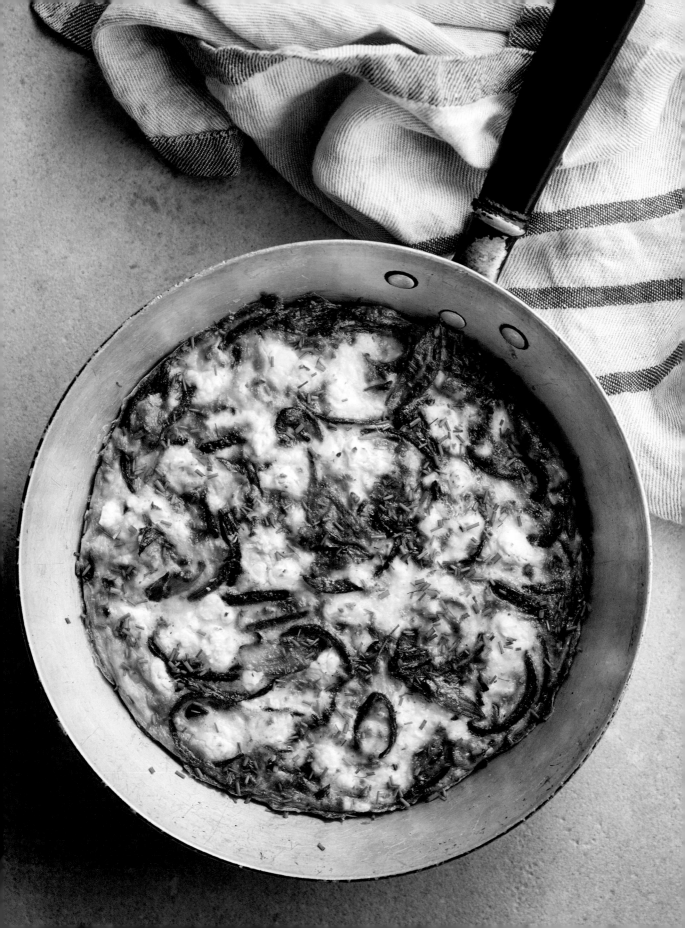

RASPBERRY POTS

PER SERVING | **215** CALS | **19G** PROTEIN | **7G** FAT | **17G** CARBS

5 MINS   1 HOUR

SERVES 2

300g low-fat Greek
  yoghurt
1/2 tsp vanilla extract
1 tsp sweetener
1/4 of a lemon
1/4 of a lime
2 digestive biscuits
20g flaxseed
100g raspberries
mint leaves, to garnish
optional: 40g low-fat
  squirty cream

*You can use a ramekin
or any glass containers
you have to hand for this
one. I freeze lemons and
limes so that I can grate
them multiple times
with less waste.*

*Who says you can't have your cake and eat it? These mini
raspberry pots taste like cheesecake – and who doesn't want
to eat cheesecake for breakfast? Cheesecake is notoriously
high in calories but these healthy pots taste just as good
without all those refined sugars, and they're only 215 calories.*

1 In a large mixing bowl, combine the yoghurt, vanilla extract
and sweetener together. Grate the lemon and lime zest into
the mixture and stir well.

2 Put the digestive biscuits into a sealable bag and crush
with a rolling pin. Divide between your containers, pressing
the crumbs firmly down into the base with the back of a spoon.
Then divide the yoghurt mixture into two and spoon over
the biscuit base.

3 Top with the flaxseed, then your raspberries, and decorate
with the mint leaves. If you have a sweet tooth, you can top
with low-fat squirty cream for an added treat. Cover and chill
in the fridge for an hour. These will keep for up to 3 days in
the fridge.

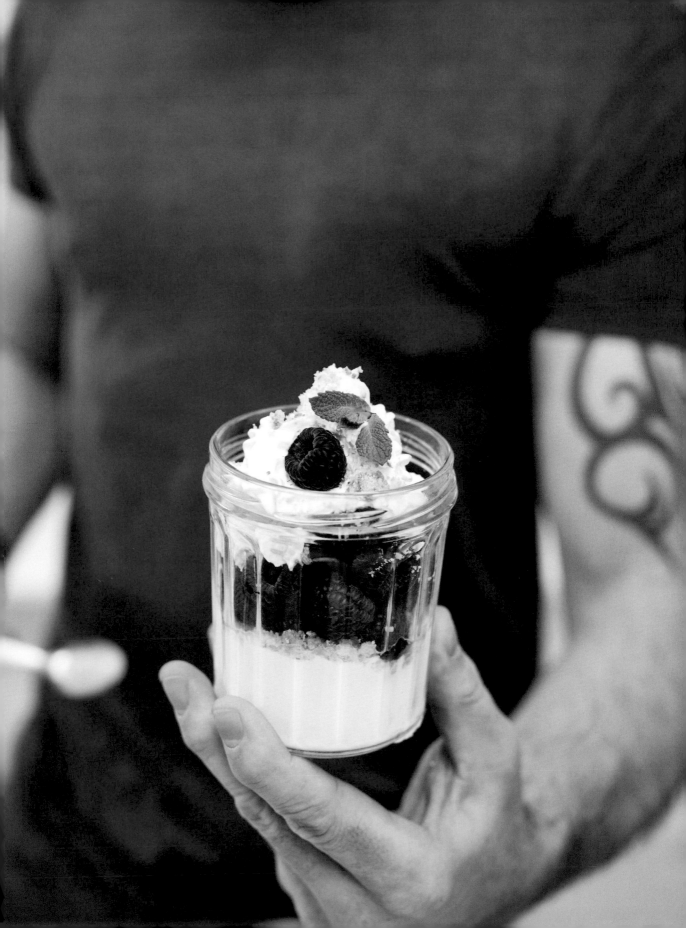

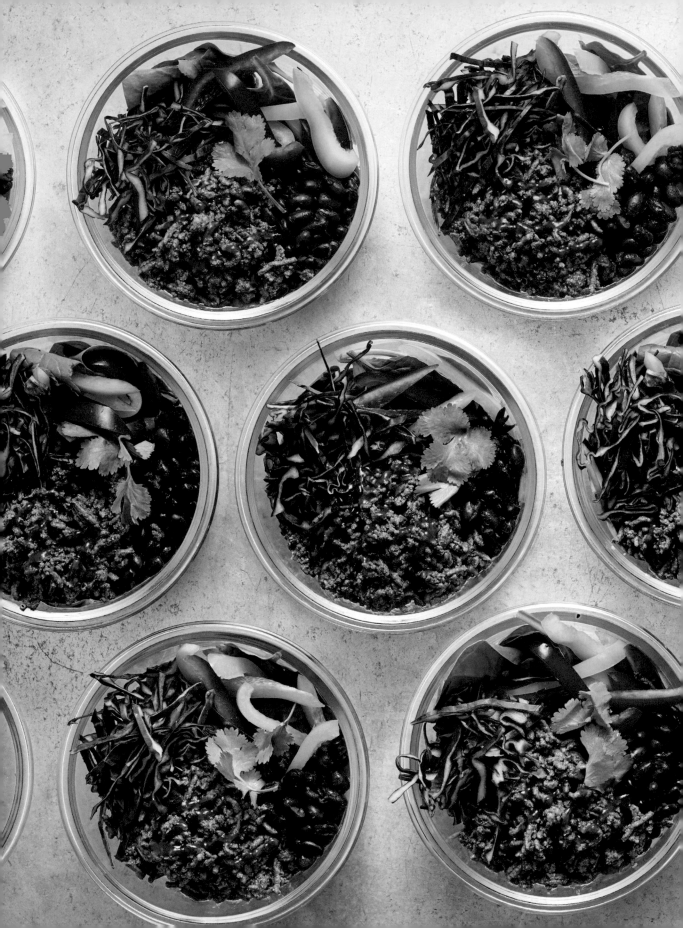

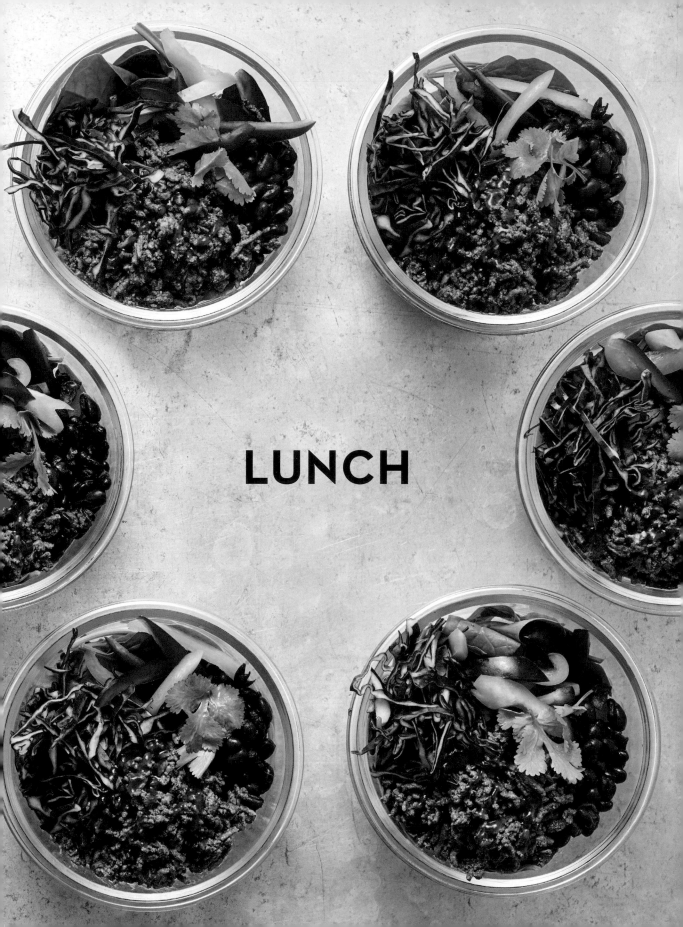

LUNCH

ROASTED RED PEPPER & TOMATO SOUP

PER SERVING | **207** CALS | **5G** PROTEIN | **13G** FAT | **15G** CARBS

15 MINS   50 MINS   FREEZE

SERVES 2

2 red peppers
300g baby plum tomatoes
1 tsp onion salt
2 tbsp olive oil
3 cloves of garlic
200g shallot onions, diced
a small bunch of fresh basil
1 bay leaf
1 chicken or vegetable
   stock cube
salt and pepper

To serve:
a swirl of single cream

A low-calorie meal prep that's delicious and healthy, plus it's easy to make. The combination of onion, peppers and tomatoes gives this soup a rich creamy flavour. It's great on its own or served with a sandwich or a salad for those extra calories.

1 Preheat the oven to 200°C. Remove the stalks from the red peppers, deseed them and cut into quarters. Then halve the tomatoes and place them all on a baking tray with the red peppers. Sprinkle with the onion salt, season and drizzle with 1 tablespoon of olive oil. Wrap the garlic cloves in foil and add them to the tray. Roast in the oven for 25–30 minutes.

2 Put the onions into a large saucepan over a medium heat with the remaining tablespoon of olive oil and sauté for 8–10 minutes until soft. Set to one side.

3 When the vegetables are ready, remove the roasted garlic from the foil and squeeze the soft cloves out of their skins into a food processor. Add the other roasted vegetables and the fried onions and blend until smooth – you will need to add 1–2 tablespoons of water to loosen it up.

4 Pour the mixture back into the saucepan used to fry the onions, add the fresh basil (whole, as it will be removed later), bay leaf, stock cube and 250ml water. Bring to the boil, then simmer for 15–20 minutes, stirring occasionally.

5 Remove the basil and bay leaf, then season to taste. The soup will keep for up to 3 days in the fridge or 3 months in the freezer. Serve with a swirl of fresh cream if you like, and it's delicious with a slice of wholegrain bread, though be sure to factor in the extra calories.

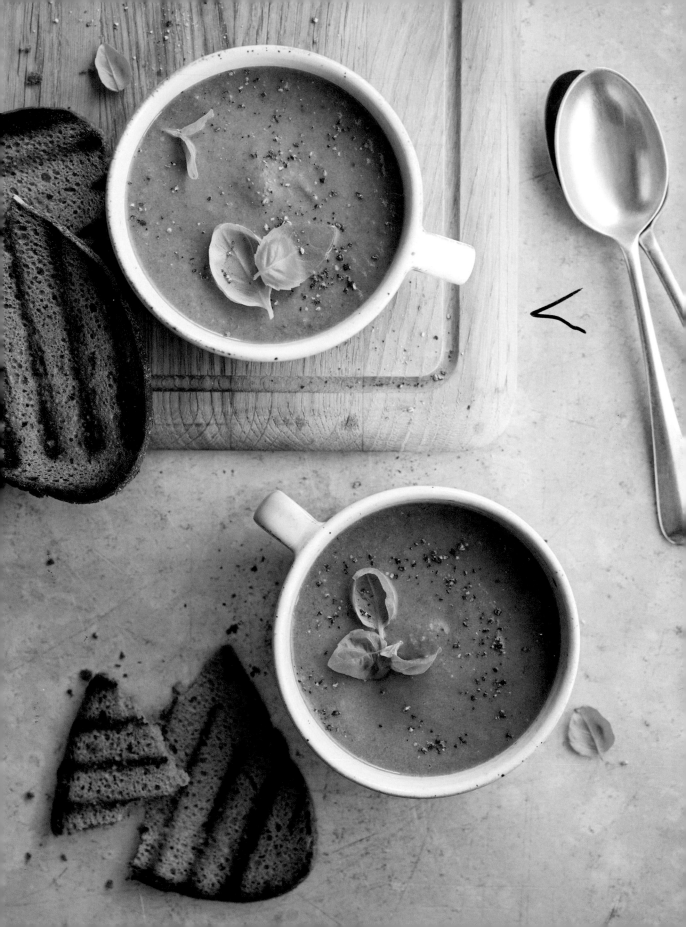

PEA, MINT & BACON SOUP

PER SERVING | **427** CALS | **24G** PROTEIN | **12G** FAT | **54G** CARBS

10 MINS   **15 MINS**   **FREEZE**

SERVES 2

200g dried marrowfat
  split peas
1 tsp bicarbonate of soda
1 onion
3 cloves of garlic, peeled
2 slices of streaky bacon
1 tbsp olive oil
1 vegetable stock cube
2 tbsp chopped mint
salt and pepper

To serve:
a swirl of cream
mint sprigs, to garnish

*If you're vegetarian, leave
out the bacon rasher.*

This delicious soup is perfect for those days when you just want that comfort feeling. It's so easy and simple to make that you'll never buy a tin of pea soup again. One of my favourite things about meal prepping soups is that you can leave them to simmer for however long you're prepping your other meals.

1 Start the night before by soaking the split peas in a large bowl with the bicarbonate of soda. The next day, make sure you rinse the peas thoroughly until you are sure all the bicarbonate of soda has been washed off.

2 Finely dice the onion, garlic and bacon. Heat the olive oil in a large saucepan over a medium heat, then sauté the onion, garlic and bacon in the pan for 8–10 minutes until they've started to soften.

3 Add the peas, the stock cube and 400ml water. Season to taste, then simmer for 5 minutes (you can simmer it for up to an hour if you wish whilst you're prepping other meals).

4 Stir in the chopped mint, check the seasoning and blend using a hand blender. This soup will keep for 3 days in the fridge or for up to 3 months in the freezer. Serve with a swirl of cream and a garnish of mint leaves, if you like.

LEEK & POTATO SOUP

PER SERVING | **487** CALS | **11G** PROTEIN | **33G** FAT | **33G** CARBS

10 MINS   40 MINS   FREEZE

SERVES 2

1 onion
2 celery stalks
1 bacon rasher
30g butter
1 tbsp olive oil
200g potatoes, peeled
200g leeks
200ml milk
1 bay leaf
1 stock cube (vegetable
   or chicken)
50g crème fraîche
salt and pepper

*If you're vegetarian, leave
out the bacon rasher.*

*This was probably one of the first recipes I ever meal
prepped. I love how you can use the full leek for a darker
soup with a fuller flavour. Alternatively, you can use just
the white part of the leek for a lighter coloured, milder
tasting soup. Both taste fantastic!*

1 Finely dice the onion, celery and bacon. Melt the butter
and oil in a large saucepan over a medium heat. Add the
onion, celery and bacon and sauté for 8–10 minutes, stirring
occasionally, until the vegetables have started to soften.

2 Whilst the vegetables are sautéing, dice the potatoes into
1cm pieces and slice the leeks. Add to the saucepan, cover
and cook for a further 10 minutes, stirring occasionally.

3 Add 200ml water, the milk, bay leaf and crumble in the
stock cube. Stir, cover again and allow to simmer for 15–20
minutes until the potato is soft (though you can simmer it
for up to an hour whilst you're making your other meals).

4 Remove the bay leaf and blend the soup with a hand
blender, then stir in the crème fraîche and season to taste.
The soup will keep for up to 3 days in the fridge or 3 months
in the freezer. It's delicious served with a slice of wholegrain
bread, though be sure to factor in the extra calories.

BUTTERNUT SQUASH SOUP

PER SERVING | **377** CALS | **5G** PROTEIN | **25G** FAT | **30G** CARBS

prep 15 MINS **cook** 50 MINS **FREEZE**

SERVES 2

1/2 a butternut squash
   (about 500g)
2 tbsp olive oil
1 carrot (about 100g)
1 onion (about 150g)
2 sticks of celery
30g butter
2 cloves of garlic,
   peeled and finely
   chopped or crushed
1 vegetable stock cube
1 bouquet garni
salt and pepper

To serve:
1 tbsp crème fraîche
chopped chives, to garnish

*It's important to stick
to the stated amount of
butter and oil used in the
recipes, otherwise you
might see your calorie
count creeping up.*

*This simple butternut squash recipe is as delicious as it's
hearty, warming and full of nutrients. Roasting the butternut
squash makes a real difference, and you can cook it in the
oven whilst prepping other meals!*

1 Preheat the oven to 200°C. Peel the squash and cut into
5cm cubes. Drizzle with 1 tablespoon of the olive oil and
season. Roast for 30–35 minutes, turning halfway, until soft.

2 Whilst the butternut squash is roasting, dice the carrot,
onion and celery. Melt the butter and the remaining tablespoon
of olive oil in a large saucepan over a medium heat. Add the
vegetables along with the garlic and sauté for 8–10 minutes,
stirring occasionally, until they begin to soften.

3 Once the butternut squash is done, add it to the other
vegetables in the saucepan and season to taste. Add a stock
cube, the bouquet garni and 400ml water, or a little more,
enough to cover the contents of the pan. Bring to the boil,
then simmer for 20–30 minutes, stirring occasionally.

4 Take the pan off the heat and remove the bouquet garni.
Then blend with a hand blender and check the seasoning.
This soup will keep for up to 3 days in the fridge or 3 months
in the freezer. To serve, add a swirl of crème fraîche and
sprinkle with finely chopped chives and black pepper.

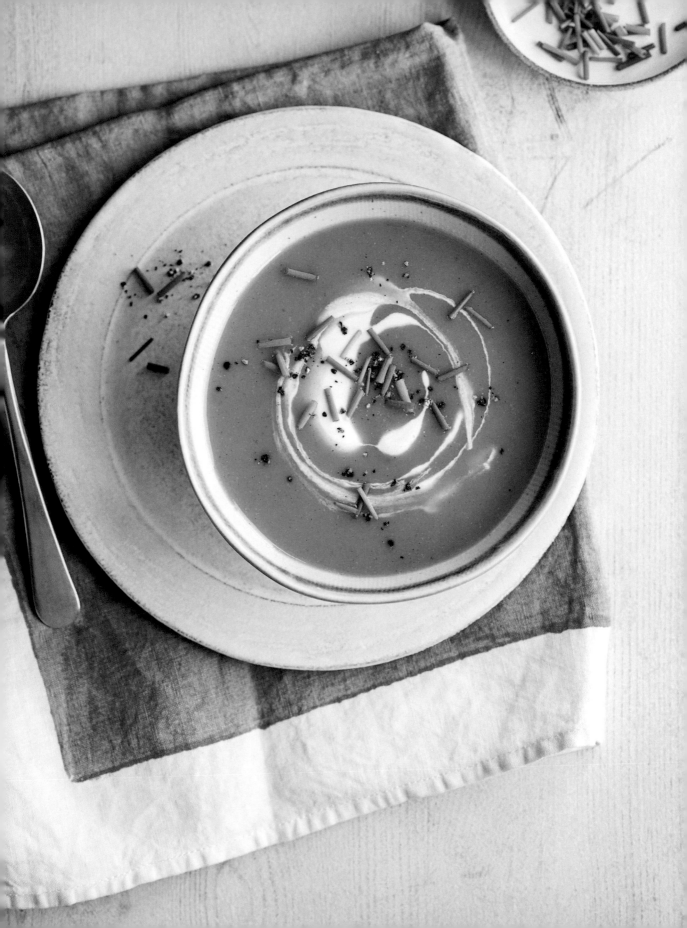

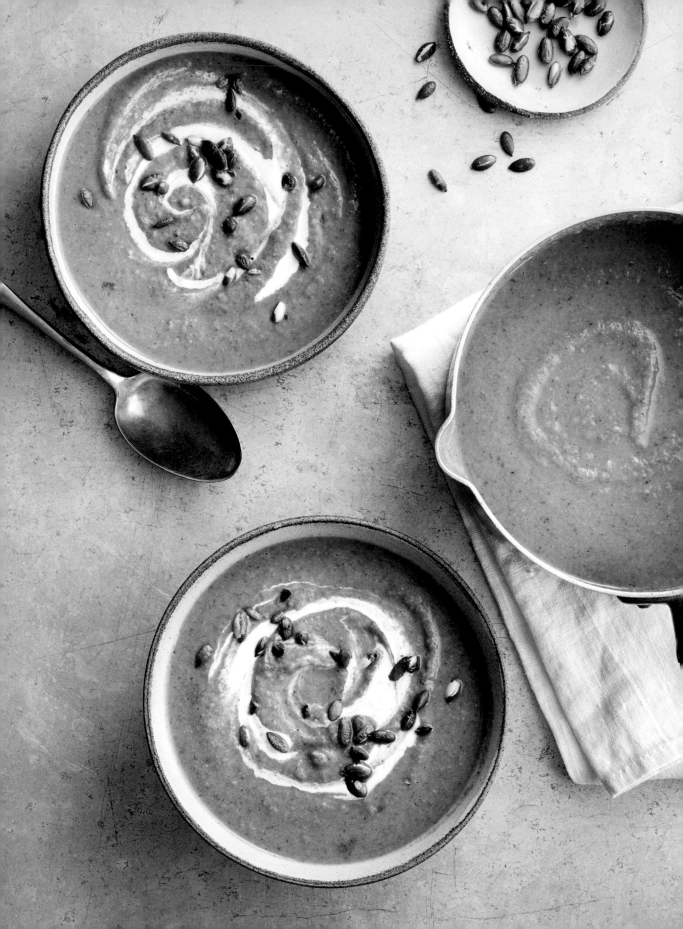

SUPER GREEN SOUP

PER SERVING | **188** CALS | **10G** PROTEIN | **8G** FAT | **14G** CARBS

5 MINS   30 MINS   FREEZE

SERVES 2

1 tbsp olive oil
1/2 an onion, diced
2 cloves of garlic, peeled
   and crushed
1/2 tsp ground turmeric
1/2 tsp ground coriander
200g frozen broccoli
   florets (or 1/2 head
   of broccoli)
50g frozen peas
50g spinach
100g winter greens
   (I use spring greens,
   kale or cavolo nero)
1 vegetable stock cube
juice of 1/2 a lemon
a small handful of fresh
   coriander leaves,
   roughly chopped
salt and pepper

To serve:
1 tbsp low-fat yoghurt
1 tsp pumpkin seeds

Eating this is bound to make you feel like a lean green machine, and it's a fantastic way of using up the vegetables in the fridge.

1 Heat the oil in a large saucepan over a medium heat and fry the onion for 8–10 minutes until soft. Add the garlic, turmeric and ground coriander, stir and fry for another minute, ensuring that it doesn't burn. Then add the broccoli florets, frozen peas, spinach, winter greens, vegetable stock cube and 500ml of water. Bring to the boil and then reduce to a simmer for 15 minutes until the vegetables are soft. Season to taste.

2 Stir through the lemon juice and the coriander leaves, then remove from the heat and blitz the soup until smooth using a hand blender. Check the seasoning and divide between two airtight containers. The soup will keep for 3 days in the fridge or for 3 months in the freezer. To serve, add some yoghurt and toasted pumpkin seeds if you like.

ROAST CHICKEN & VEGETABLE TRAYBAKE

PER SERVING | **460** CALS | **27G** PROTEIN | **24G** FAT | **30G** CARBS

10 MINS   45 MINS

SERVES 2

1 sweet potato
   (approx. 250g)
100g broccoli
1/2 a small red onion
1 courgette
4 cloves of garlic
2 chicken thigh fillets
   (approx. 250g)
2 tbsp olive oil
3 sprigs of fresh thyme
salt and pepper

The thing I love about this meal prep is that everything goes on one tray in the oven and cooks whilst you prep other meals. It's also great for using up any vegetables I have left in the fridge. To keep the cost down, use seasonal vegetables.

1 Preheat the oven to 200°C. Then start prepping the vegetables: chop the sweet potato into 3cm cubes, break the broccoli up into florets, slice the onion into four wedges and halve the courgette and cut it into bite-sized pieces. Put the chopped vegetables into a large non-stick baking tray along with the whole garlic cloves.

2 Add the chicken thigh fillets to the tray and sprinkle a little salt over the top. Drizzle over the olive oil, season with salt and pepper and add the sprigs of thyme.

3 Oven roast for 40–45 minutes, turning the vegetables halfway, until the chicken is fully cooked and the vegetables are tender. You can eat it straight away or divide it between two airtight containers. It will keep in the fridge for 3 days or in the freezer for up to 3 months.

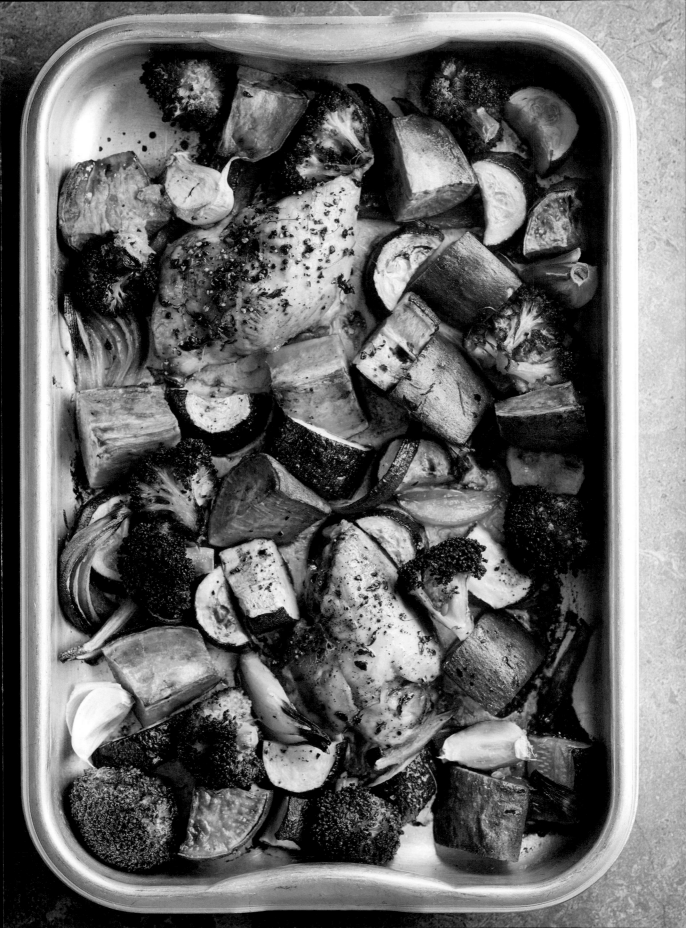

JACKET POTATO WITH PORK & BBQ BEANS

PER SERVING | **496** CALS | **25G** PROTEIN | **14G** FAT | **62G** CARBS

prep **cook** **FREEZE**
10 MINS 40 MINS

SERVES 2

2 jacket potatoes
   (150g each)
low-cal spray oil
salt
1 onion, peeled
2 garlic cloves, peeled
1 bacon rasher
1 pork medallion
1 tbsp olive oil
1 x 400g tin of haricot
   beans, drained
150g passata
1 tbsp tomato purée
1/4 tsp mustard powder
1/4 tsp ground allspice
1/4 tsp chilli powder
1 tsp light soy sauce
10g brown sugar

These BBQ beans are a real game changer. Traditional baked beans are well known for containing huge amounts of salt and sugar but by making them yourself you can control the amount that goes into them. Not to mention they taste fantastic. Well worth that little bit of effort!

1 Preheat the oven to 200°C. Stab each jacket potato with a fork a few times, then microwave each one for 6–8 minutes. Remove from the microwave, spray with the low-cal oil, sprinkle with salt and place in a roasting tin in the oven for 30 minutes, turning halfway, until golden and cooked through. Set to one side.

2 Whilst the potatoes are baking, finely dice the onion, garlic and bacon, then slice the pork medallion into thin strips.

3 Heat the olive oil in a medium-sized frying pan over a medium heat. Sauté the onion, garlic and bacon for 8–10 minutes until they've softened. Then add the thinly sliced pork and cook for a further 2–3 minutes. Pour in the haricot beans, passata, tomato purée, spices, soy sauce, sugar and 50ml water and mix well. Simmer for 10–15 minutes until the sauce has thickened.

4 These will keep in the fridge for up to 3 days or in the freezer for up to 3 months. Serve with a side salad (store in a separate container if prepared in advance).

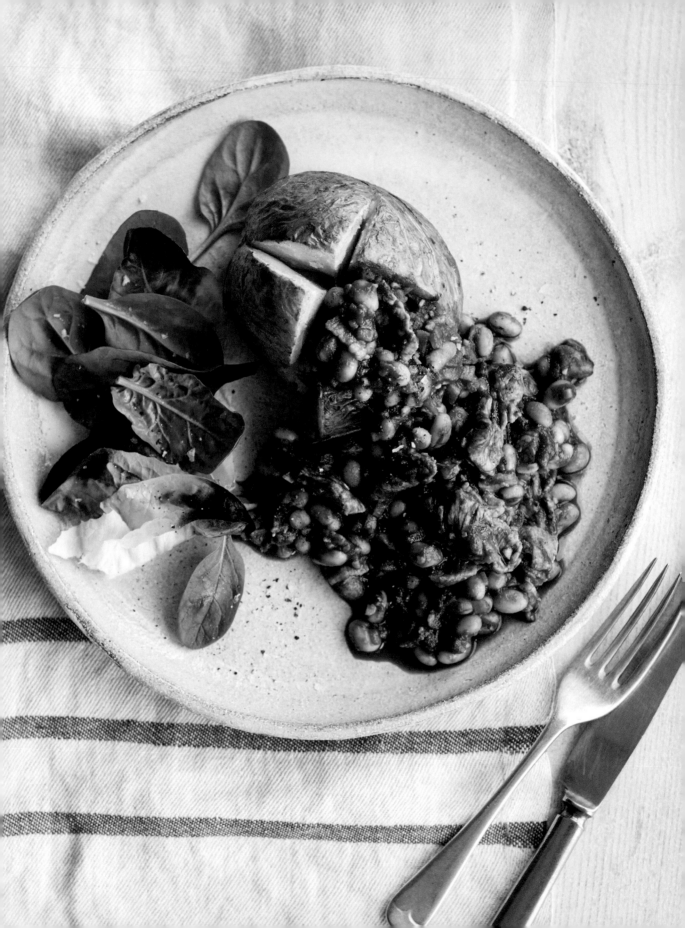

MEXICAN BEEF BURRITO BOWLS

PER SERVING | **451** CALS | **48G** PROTEIN | **14G** FAT | **29G** CARBS

5 MINS   10 MINS   FREEZE

SERVES 2

1 tbsp olive oil
330g lean minced beef
1 x 400g tin of black beans,
   drained and rinsed
2 peppers, finely sliced
a few sprigs of fresh
   coriander, leaves picked
   and finely chopped
salt and pepper

*For the Mexican seasoning
(or use a ready-made taco
mix, to taste):*
1/2 tsp chilli powder
1/4 tsp garlic powder
1/4 tsp dried oregano
1/2 tsp paprika
2/3 tsp ground cumin

To serve:
20g red cabbage,
   thinly sliced
a handful of baby
   spinach leaves
a drizzle of sriracha

Swapping out your taco shell or tortilla for black beans is a fantastic way of getting extra fibre and protein into your diet. This healthy lunch is quick to make as well as filling – the perfect combination.

1 Heat the olive oil in a frying pan over a medium heat until hot. Add the beef in batches so it browns evenly and fry for 5–8 minutes, stirring occasionally.

2 Combine the spices in a bowl and mix them into the mince just before you finish frying it. Remove from the heat and season to taste.

3 Divide the black beans and sliced peppers between two airtight containers. Split the mince mix between the containers and top with the coriander leaves. If you want to spice things up, you can garnish with thinly sliced red cabbage, baby spinach leaves and a drizzle of sriracha. The meals will keep for 3 days in the fridge or up to 3 months in the freezer.

Sprinkle a little bit of water over the mince before reheating to avoid it drying out.

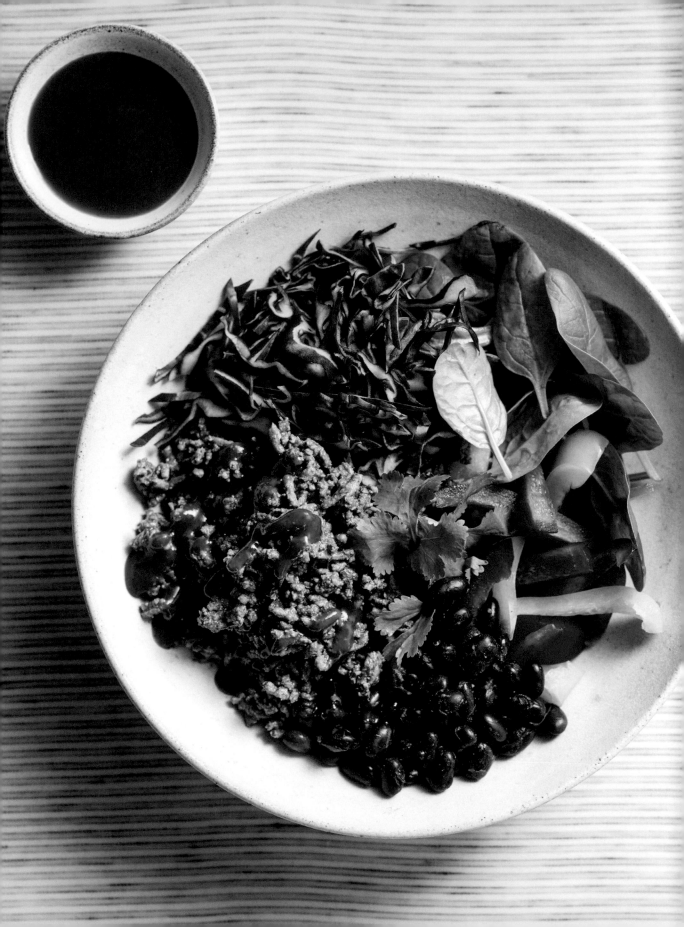

CHICKEN FAJITA BOWLS

PER SERVING | **499** CALS | **37G** PROTEIN | **20G** FAT | **41G** CARBS

prep 10 MINS **cook** 40 MINS **FREEZE**

SERVES 2

300g skinless, boneless
   chicken thighs
1 pepper
1 red onion, peeled
low-cal spray oil
100g wholegrain rice
40g low-fat Cheddar
   cheese, grated
a handful of fresh flat-leaf
   parsley, roughly chopped

*For the fajita seasoning
(or use a ready-made
mix, to taste):*
1/2 tsp chilli powder (adjust
   the amount according
   to your heat tolerance)
1/2 tbsp smoked paprika
a pinch of ground cumin
1/2 tsp garlic powder
1/2 tsp dried oregano
a pinch of onion powder
a pinch of cayenne pepper

*This simple and super-quick meal prep is pretty much
all done in the oven, which makes it a firm Meal Prep King
favourite. You won't go far wrong with this really simple
recipe and it's great to have on the go whilst cooking
other things – a multi-task must!*

1 Preheat the oven to 200°C. Cut the chicken thighs and
pepper into strips, then finely slice the onion. Put it all into
a large mixing bowl and spray in a good amount of low-cal
oil. Then mix in the fajita seasoning.

2 Put the chicken, peppers and onions on a baking tray, spreading
them out to ensure even cooking. Cook for 35–40 minutes in
the centre of the oven or until the chicken is cooked through.

3 Meanwhile, cook the rice according to the packet
instructions and divide between two airtight containers.
Top the rice with the cooked chicken mix.

4 Once the fajitas have cooled, sprinkle with some cheese
and parsley. When the meal is reheated this will melt together
and taste delicious. The fajitas will keep in the fridge for up
to 1 day or in the freezer for up to 3 months.

 tips

*Add a wedge of lime and squeeze over the meal after it's been
reheated, as it will bring the freshness back to life. You can freeze
the meal without the rice.*

*It's best to freeze or refrigerate rice as soon as possible after
cooking it, once it's cooled down. It'll keep in the fridge for up
to 1 day. When reheating, make sure it is steaming hot all the
way through. Do not reheat cooked rice more than once.*

PESTO CHICKEN

PER SERVING | **400** CALS | **44G** PROTEIN | **22G** FAT | **4G** CARBS

5 MINS   30 MINS

SERVES 2

2 chicken breasts
2 tbsp green pesto
1 tomato, sliced
125g mozzarella
200g tenderstem broccoli
juice of ½ a lemon
salt and pepper

You can cook the chicken as per the method opposite and it will keep in the freezer for up to 3 months. When you reheat it, all you'll have to do is cook the broccoli to go with it.

You can use your own homemade pesto for this succulent chicken recipe or you can cheat with some shop-bought pesto. Either way, it's a tasty meal and preps an absolute treat!

1 Preheat the oven to 200°C and line a baking tray with baking paper. Put the chicken breasts between two sheets of baking paper or clingfilm and bash with a rolling pin until they are the same thickness all over (this ensures even cooking). Place the chicken on the lined baking tray and spread the pesto evenly over each one, then top with the sliced tomato and mozzarella. Bake in the oven for 25–30 minutes until the chicken is cooked through (you can check this by poking a knife into it: if the juices run clear, then it's cooked).

2 Whilst the chicken is baking, bring a saucepan of water to the boil and cook the tenderstem broccoli for 1–2 minutes. Remove with a slotted spoon and plunge into ice-cold water, then drain.

3 Divide the broccoli between two airtight containers, squeeze over the lemon juice and season. Top with the pesto chicken. It will keep in the fridge for up to 3 days.

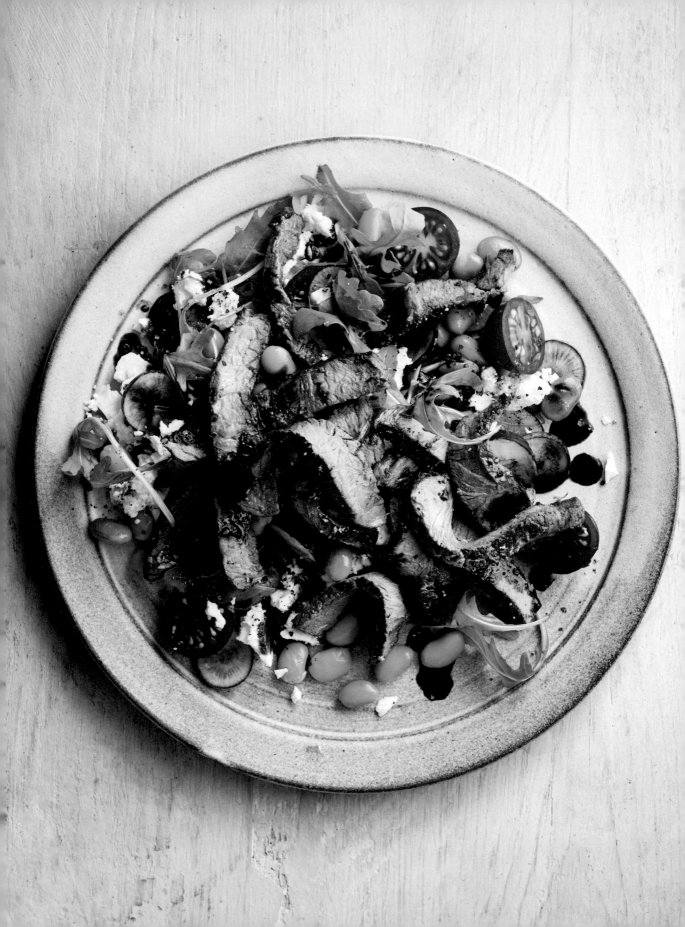

BALSAMIC STEAK & FETA CHEESE SALAD WITH EDAMAME BEANS

PER SERVING | **424** CALS | **35G** PROTEIN | **26G** FAT | **11G** CARBS

10 MINS   10 MINS
+
MARINATING

SERVES 2

1 clove of garlic,
    finely chopped
20ml balsamic vinegar
3 sprigs of fresh thyme,
    leaves picked
1 tbsp olive oil
1 rump steak
40g rocket
50g feta cheese
100g cherry tomatoes,
    halved
100g edamame beans
40g radishes, sliced
optional: a drizzle of
    balsamic glaze
salt and pepper

*For best results, try
to marinate the meat
overnight, or at least for
a few hours beforehand.
It takes around 8 hours
for the steaks to take
on maximum flavour.*

Steak goes with almost anything, so don't be afraid to use whatever you already have to save on waste, though do keep the calories in mind!

1 Place the garlic, balsamic vinegar, thyme, half a tablespoon of the olive oil and seasoning in a bowl and mix together. Cover the steak in the mixture, rubbing it in thoroughly so that the meat is fully coated. Place in an airtight container and leave in the fridge overnight.

2 Take your steak out of the fridge 15 minutes before you plan on cooking it so it comes up to room temperature. Heat the remaining olive oil in a frying pan over a high heat and add any leftover thyme you may have, and some more garlic if you wish. Cook the steak how you like it: $1^{1}/_{2}$ minutes on each side for rare, $2^{1}/_{2}$ minutes on each side for medium and 4–5 minutes on each side for well done. Allow to rest for 5–10 minutes after cooking.

3 Divide the rocket between two airtight containers, then crumble in the feta cheese and add the cherry tomatoes, edamame beans and radishes.

4 Slice the steak up into strips and enjoy warm or allow to cool before adding to your meal prep boxes – this will ensure your salad doesn't get ruined by the heat of the steak. Drizzle over some balsamic glaze, if you like, and enjoy. This salad will keep for up to 3 days in the fridge.

CHORIZO & FETA SALAD WITH RED PEPPER DRESSING

PER SERVING | **460** CALS | **20G** PROTEIN | **23G** FAT | **40G** CARBS

10 MINS   40 MINS

SERVES 2

60g chorizo sausage
50g kale
40g rocket
60g feta cheese

For the dressing:
200g sweet pointed
  pepper
1 tbsp olive oil
10g honey
1 clove of garlic, peeled
20ml apple cider vinegar
a few sprigs of fresh parsley
a few sprigs of fresh basil
salt and pepper

To serve:
2 wholemeal pitta breads

I created this recipe using only the leftover ingredients I had in the fridge. Who knew that something so simple could taste so good – especially the dressing! It's now a weekly recipe in the Meal Prep King's household.

1 To make the dressing, preheat the oven to 200°C. Deseed the sweet peppers and chop into 5cm cubes. Place the peppers on a baking tray, drizzle with the olive oil and season. Roast for 25–30 minutes until tender.

2 Once the sweet peppers are ready, put them in a food processor along with the honey, garlic, apple cider vinegar and 3–5 tablespoons of water. Blend until smooth. Coarsely chop the parsley and basil (leaves and stalks) and add to the dressing. Check the seasoning and set to one side.

3 Dice the chorizo sausage into 5mm pieces and add to a dry pan over a medium heat. Fry for about 1–2 minutes until you see the oil coming out. Then steam the kale for about 30 seconds–1 minute (you can also do this in the microwave – check the packet for instructions); be sure to add 1–2 tablespoons of water to the bowl when you do so.

4 Put the rocket and kale into two airtight containers, crumble in the feta cheese and add the chorizo. Drizzle the juices from the pan over the salad (you won't regret it!).

5 Put your red pepper dressing into a separate container unless you are eating the salad immediately. The salad will keep in the fridge for up to 3 days. Serve with warm wholemeal pitta breads if you like.

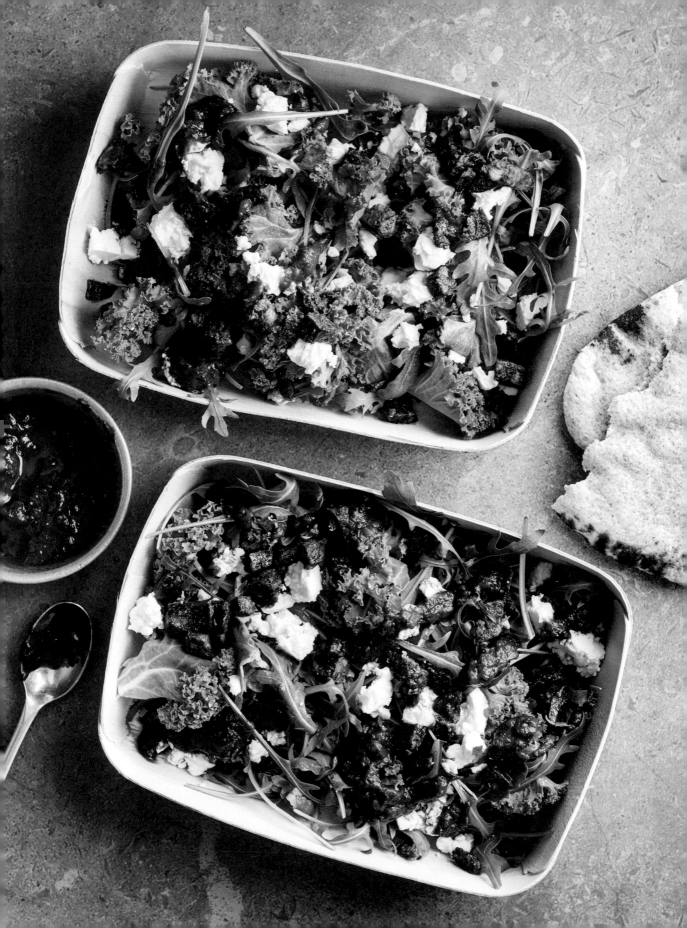

TURMERIC CHICKEN WITH RICE & GREENS

PER SERVING | **453** CALS | **38G** PROTEIN | **9G** FAT | **52G** CARBS

10 MINS   25 MINS
+
MARINATING

SERVES 2

2 chicken breasts
2 tsp ground turmeric
1 tsp garlic salt
1 tsp onion granules
1 tbsp olive oil
juice of 1/2 a lemon
120g rice
200g tenderstem broccoli
1 yellow courgette,
   peeled into strips
salt and pepper

You can cook the chicken as per the method and it will keep in the freezer for up to 3 months. When you reheat it, all you'll have to do is cook the rice, broccoli and courgette to go with it.

It's best to freeze or refrigerate rice as soon as possible after cooking it, once it's cooled down. It'll keep in the fridge for up to 1 day. When reheating, make sure it is steaming hot all the way through. Do not reheat cooked rice more than once.

This is a great way to introduce turmeric into your everyday cooking. Not only does it taste great but turmeric also has a whole range of health benefits. This is a quick and easy recipe that will leave your taste buds wanting more.

1 Preheat the oven to 200°C. Put the chicken breasts between two sheets of baking paper or clingfilm and bash with a rolling pin until they are the same thickness all over (this ensures even cooking). Then place the chicken breasts in an airtight container or a ziplock food bag with the spices, olive oil and lemon juice and seasoning. Leave to marinate in the fridge for 2 hours before cooking or overnight if possible.

2 Heat a frying pan over a high heat and fry the chicken breasts for 1 minute on either side until sealed. Then wrap the chicken in foil and bake in the oven for 20–25 minutes. Cut the cooked chicken into bite-sized slices.

3 Whilst the chicken is baking, cook the rice according to the packet instructions. Bring a saucepan of water to the boil and cook the tenderstem broccoli for 1–2 minutes. Remove with a slotted spoon and plunge into ice-cold water, then drain.

4 Divide the rice, tenderstem broccoli and yellow courgette strips between two airtight containers and top each one with the chicken slices. This meal will keep in the fridge for up to 1 day.

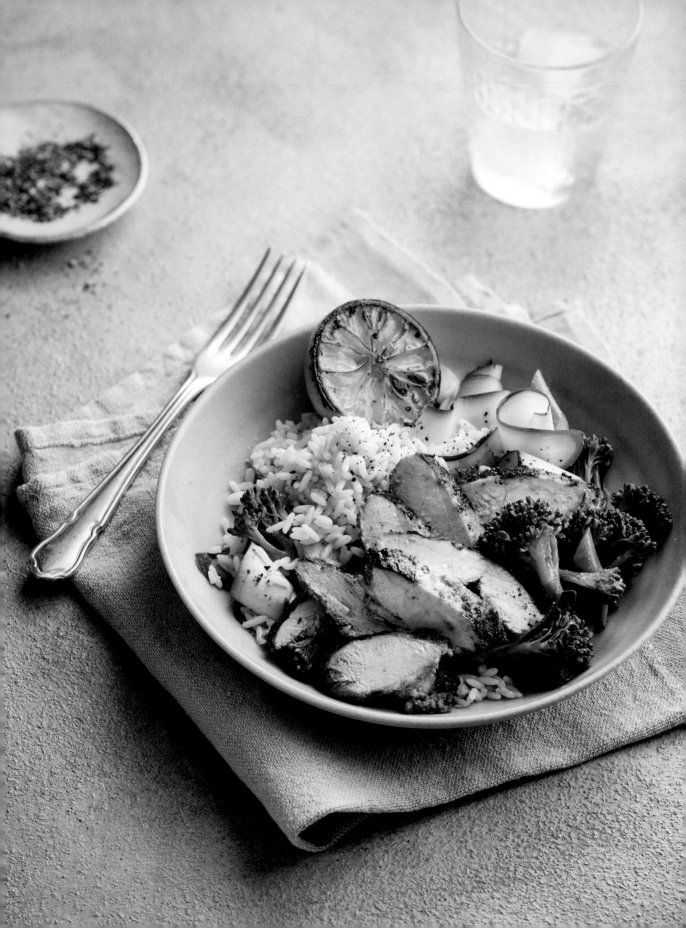

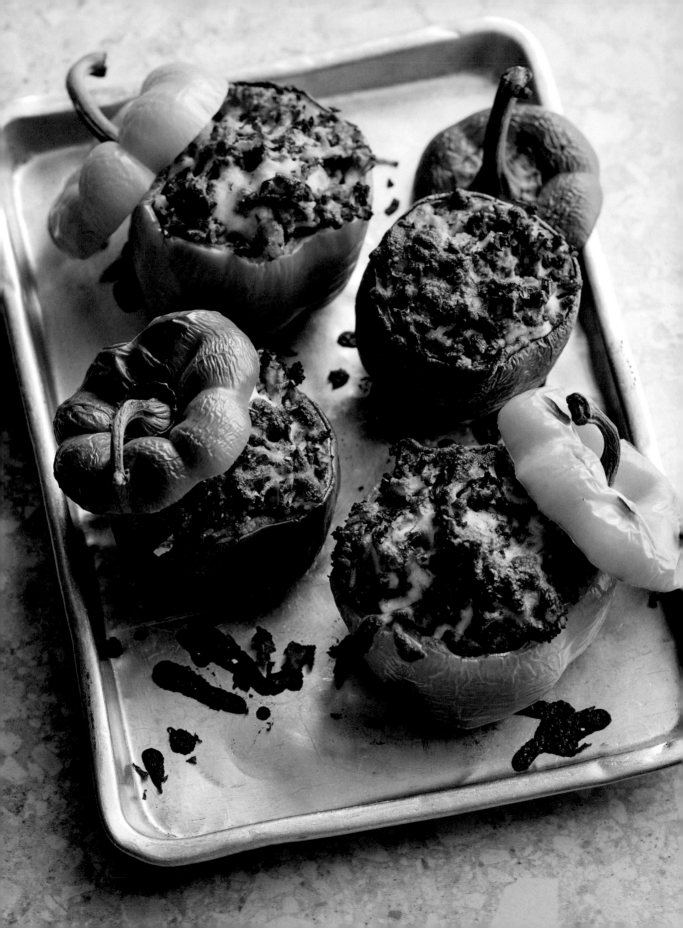

TURKEY-STUFFED PEPPERS

PER SERVING | 393 CALS | 41G PROTEIN | 16G FAT | 19G CARBS

10 MINS   40 MINS   FREEZE

SERVES 2

2 peppers (any colour)
1 tbsp olive oil
250g turkey mince
1/2 an onion, peeled and diced
1 clove of garlic, finely chopped
50g passata
60g precooked white rice
   or quinoa
20g low-fat mozzarella
   cheese, shredded
a handful of fresh parsley,
   roughly chopped
salt and pepper

*For the chilli spice mix (or use
a ready-made mix, to taste):*
1/4 tsp chilli powder (adjust
   the amount according
   to your heat tolerance)
1/2 tsp smoked paprika
1/4 tsp ground cumin
1/4 tsp garlic powder
1/4 tsp dried oregano
1/4 tsp ground coriander
1/4 tsp black pepper
1/4 tsp ground fenugreek

*It's best to freeze or
refrigerate rice as soon as
possible after cooking it,
once it's cooled down. It'll
keep in the fridge for up
to 1 day. When reheating,
make sure it is steaming
hot all the way through.
Do not reheat cooked
rice more than once.*

*This is a colourful and vibrant dish that reheats brilliantly,
which makes it an ideal addition to any weekly meal prep.
Serve with a side of any leftover vegetables you have kicking
around in the fridge to pack in some extra nutrients.*

1 Preheat the oven to 220°C. Chop off the tops of the
peppers and remove the seeds and white flesh. Stand them
up on a baking tray (if they won't stand up, cut a sliver off
the bottom so that they will). Cover with foil and cook in
the oven for 20 minutes.

2 Meanwhile, put half a tablespoon of the olive oil into
a frying pan over a medium heat. Add the mince to the pan
in small batches so it browns nicely. Fry for 6–8 minutes until
cooked. Remove the mince from the pan and set aside. Use
the same pan to fry the onion and garlic with half a tablespoon
of olive oil for 8–10 minutes, or until they start to soften.

3 Add the spice mix, the passata and the cooked rice or
quinoa, then season to taste and mix well.

4 Stuff each roasted pepper with the mixture. If you're eating
right away, top them with cheese and parsley and put them
back in the oven for 15–20 minutes until the cheese is golden.
If you are using these for meal prep, allow the peppers to cool,
cut them in half, then top with cheese – this will melt when
you come to reheat them. These will keep in the fridge for
up to 1 day or in the freezer for up to 3 months. Serve with
a handful of fresh salad if you like.

KOREAN-STYLE BEEF NOODLES

PER SERVING | **398** CALS | **34G** PROTEIN | **7G** FAT | **47G** CARBS

10 MINS   15 MINS   FREEZE

SERVES 2

225g lean rump steak
low-cal spray oil
20g honey
½ tsp hot chilli sauce
2 tbsp soy sauce
1 tsp rice vinegar
1 tsp crushed garlic
1 tsp cornflour
140g spring greens
100g wholegrain noodles
salt and pepper

Optional toppings:
2 spring onions, sliced
1 tsp sesame seeds
½ a red chilli, sliced

An Asian-inspired recipe that's a healthy take on comfort food. You can get it on the table or into a meal prep container in under 30 minutes – less time than it takes to order a takeaway!

1 Let the beef get to room temperature for 20–30 minutes, then slice into bite-sized chunks. Heat a frying pan over a high heat and spray the pan with low-cal oil. Fry the beef for 2 minutes, turning halfway through, then remove and set aside.

2 Lower the heat to medium and add the honey, chilli sauce, soy sauce, rice vinegar and garlic to the frying pan. Deglaze the pan by scraping the browned bits off the bottom of the pan, then whisk the cornflour and 2–3 tablespoons of water together to form a paste before adding to the pan.

3 Once the sauce has thickened, add the steak and cook until it's done to your liking. Meanwhile, steam the spring greens for 6–8 minutes and cook the noodles according to the packet instructions.

4 Remove the cooked beef from the sauce and set aside. Add the drained noodles to the sauce and stir, ensuring that the noodles are fully coated in the sauce. Divide the spring greens and noodles between two airtight containers, then top with the cooked beef. If you wish, garnish with sliced spring onion, sesame seeds and sliced chilli. This meal will keep in the fridge for up to 3 days or in the freezer for up to 3 months.

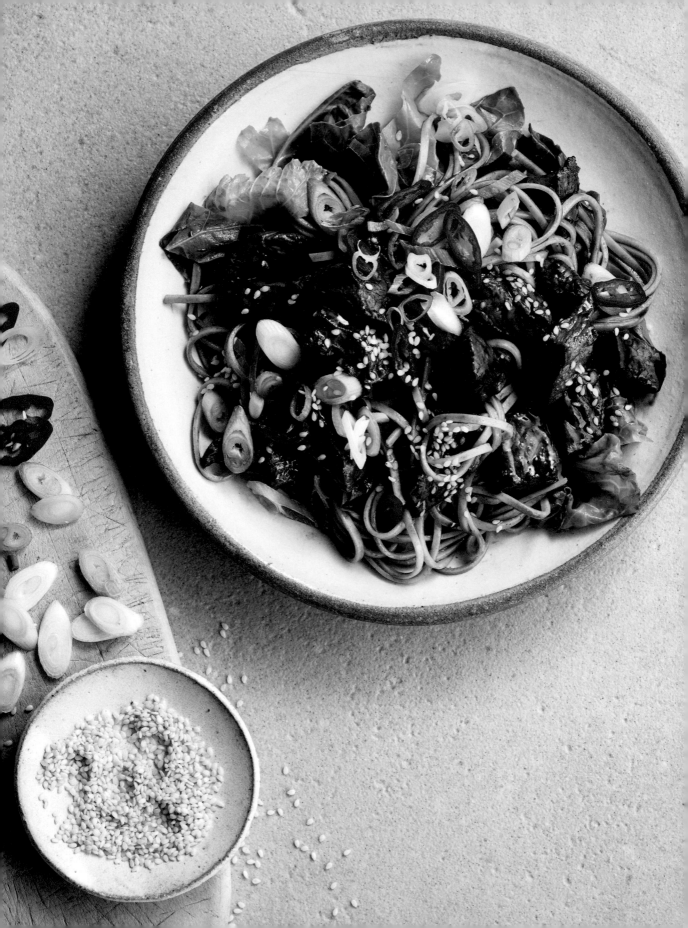

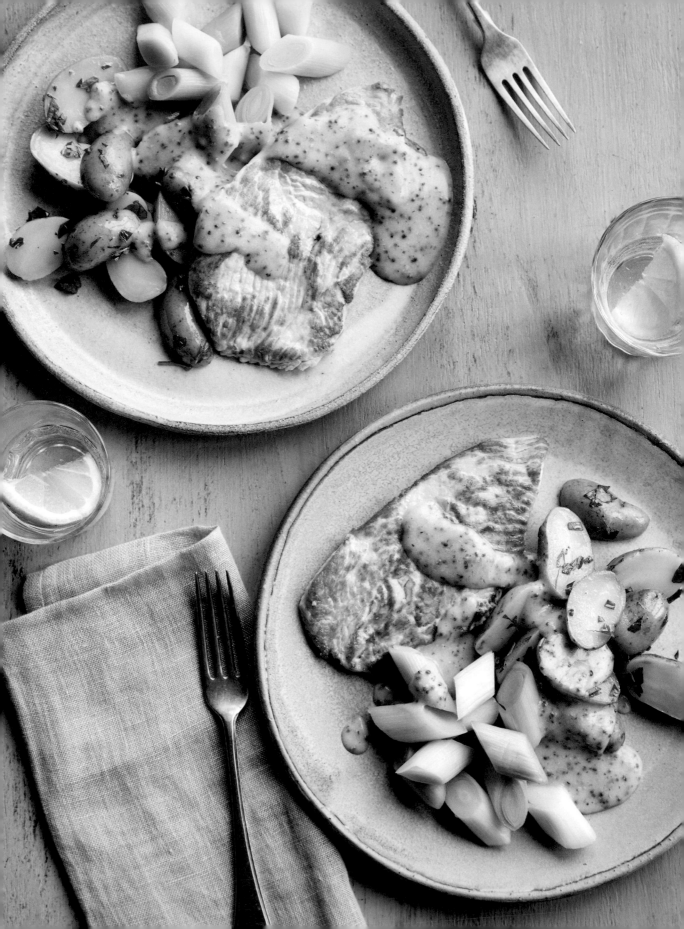

TURKEY STEAKS WITH NEW POTATOES, STEAMED LEEKS & MUSTARD SAUCE

PER SERVING | **341** CALS | **36G** PROTEIN | **11G** FAT | **23G** CARBS

5 MINS   20 MINS   FREEZE

SERVES 2

200g new potatoes
100g leeks
1 tbsp olive oil
2 turkey breast steaks

For the sauce:
10g low-fat margarine
1 tbsp plain flour
150ml skimmed milk
1 tbsp wholegrain mustard
salt and pepper

What could be simpler than pan-fried turkey steak with steamed vegetables and potatoes? If you're meal prepping this, store the mustard sauce separately from the meal and simply pour over the steaks and potatoes when you're ready to eat.

1 Halve the new potatoes and slice the leeks. Place the potatoes in a pan of water and bring to the boil. Boil for 15 minutes until tender. Five minutes before they'll be ready, place a steamer on top of the pan and steam the leeks. (If you don't have a steamer, add the leeks to the pan with the potatoes for the last 3 minutes.)

2 Heat the oil in a frying pan over a medium heat. Add the turkey steaks to the pan and fry them for 3–4 minutes, turning once, until golden brown and cooked.

3 Meanwhile, melt the margarine in a saucepan over a medium-to-low heat. Once it's melted, add the flour and whisk for 1–2 minutes until a roux forms (it should be smooth and pale). Pour the milk in, a little at a time, whisking continuously until you have a smooth sauce. Leave it to thicken on a low heat for 5 minutes, then stir in the mustard and season to taste.

4 If you're eating straight away, divide the vegetables between two plates, top with a turkey steak and drizzle over the mustard sauce. If you're meal prepping it, divide the vegetables and turkey steaks between two airtight containers. Divide the mustard sauce between two small pots. This meal will keep in the fridge for up to 3 days or in the freezer for up to 3 weeks.

MEDITERRANEAN CHICKEN KEBABS WITH A HERBY DIP

PER SERVING | **273 CALS** | **35G PROTEIN** | **9G FAT** | **12G CARBS**

15 MINS 20 MINS FREEZE

SERVES 2

2 chicken breasts
1 red onion, peeled
1 pepper (any colour),
    deseeded
80g mixed salad leaves

For the marinade:
1 tbsp olive oil
juice of 1/2 a lemon
1/2 tsp dried marjoram
1/2 tsp dried sage
1/2 tsp dried thyme
1/2 tsp dried basil
1 tsp paprika
1/2 tsp garlic powder
a pinch of black pepper
a pinch of chilli flakes
a pinch of sea salt

For the herby dip:
a handful of fresh herbs
    (I suggest basil, chives,
    parsley or dill)
100g low-fat Greek yoghurt
1/2 tbsp white wine vinegar
juice of 1/2 a lemon
salt and pepper

To serve:
mini flatbreads

Chicken kebab, anyone? This is a recipe that can be enjoyed either hot or cold. Succulent and fragrant chicken accompanied by a light and fresh dip – delicious!

1 Cut the chicken breasts into bite-sized pieces and put them in an airtight container. Then chop the onion into wedges and the pepper into 5cm pieces and add them too. Mix the marinade ingredients together, pour into the container and mix to ensure the chicken and vegetables are thoroughly coated, then leave to marinate for an hour in the fridge.

2 If using wooden skewers, pre-soak them in water to stop them burning when under the grill.

3 To make the herby dip, finely chop the fresh herbs and mix well with the yoghurt, white wine vinegar and lemon juice. Season to taste.

4 Add the chicken pieces to the skewers one at a time, adding onion wedges and pepper chunks in sequence until all the meat and vegetables are used up. Grill under a medium heat for 15–20 minutes, turning after 10 minutes. You can serve these just as they are with the salad leaves or add some mini flatbreads (but remember to add the calories). The kebabs will keep in the fridge for up to 3 days or in the freezer (minus the dip) for up to 3 months.

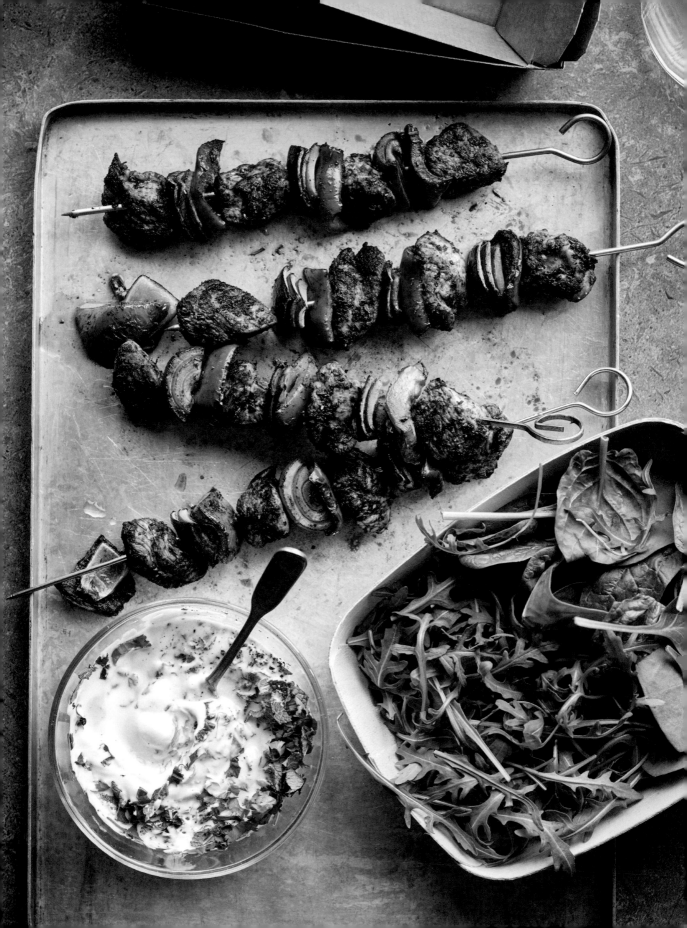

CHICKEN CAESAR SALAD

PER SERVING | **403** CALS | **45G** PROTEIN | **14G** FAT | **24G** CARBS

10 MINS 30 MINS

SERVES 2

2 slices of white bread
1 tsp mixed herbs
1 tbsp olive oil
2 chicken breasts
1/2 a head of lettuce,
    leaves separated
    and roughly torn
salt and pepper

For the dressing:
1/2 a clove of garlic,
    peeled and crushed
4 tbsp low-fat Greek
    yoghurt
juice of 1/2 a lemon
1 tsp Worcestershire sauce
2 anchovies, finely sliced
15g Parmesan cheese,
    grated
1 tbsp white wine vinegar

A great recipe for using up any leftover bread! Cooking the chicken in foil is a great way of ensuring that it's succulent and juicy.

1 Preheat the oven to 200°C. Tear up the slices of bread and scatter over a baking tray. Sprinkle over the mixed herbs, drizzle over the olive oil, season and mix, making sure the olive oil has coated all the bread. Bake for 8–10 minutes, turning the croutons over occasionally, until golden brown.

2 Season the chicken breasts and wrap them in foil. Bake in the oven for 20–25 minutes, until the juices run clear when you poke a knife into the meat, then take them out and cut into bite-sized strips.

3 Divide the lettuce leaves, chicken and croutons between two airtight containers. Mix all the dressing ingredients together and season to taste. Split the dressing between two small pots and put into the containers. This meal will keep in the fridge for up to 3 days.

BAKED FALAFEL WITH COUSCOUS SALAD & TAHINI DRESSING

PER SERVING | **493** CALS | **21G** PROTEIN | **14G** FAT | **65G** CARBS

prep   *cook*

10 MINS   30 MINS

SERVES 2

low-cal spray oil
1 x 400g tin of chickpeas, drained
1/2 tsp ground cumin
1/2 tsp ground coriander
1/2 tsp paprika
1/2 tsp garlic powder
1/2 tsp onion granules
a small handful of fresh coriander, roughly chopped
1 tbsp flour
juice of 1 lemon
100g couscous
1 tomato, diced
1/2 a cucumber, diced
salt and pepper

For the dressing:
30g tahini
juice of 1 lemon

You can freeze the cooked falafel, if you want to make them ahead. They will keep for up to 3 months.

Falafel are delicious and baking them is a much healthier way of cooking them than the usual frying! I serve them with a couscous salad and tahini dressing, which are packed full of flavour.

1 Preheat the oven to 200°C, then line a baking tray with baking paper and spritz with low-cal oil. Put the chickpeas, cumin, ground coriander, paprika, garlic powder, onion granules and fresh coriander into a food processor and blitz until smooth. Season to taste.

2 Stir in the flour and lemon juice. Mould the mixture into eight patties, place them on the baking tray and bake for 25–30 minutes, flipping them over halfway through, until golden brown.

3 Whilst the falafels are baking, cook the couscous according to the packet instructions. Drain, then mix in the diced tomato and cucumber and season to taste.

4 Whisk the tahini, lemon juice and 25ml cold water together to create the dressing. Divide the couscous salad between two airtight containers and add four falafels to each. Split the dressing between two small pots and add to the containers. This will keep in the fridge for up to 3 days.

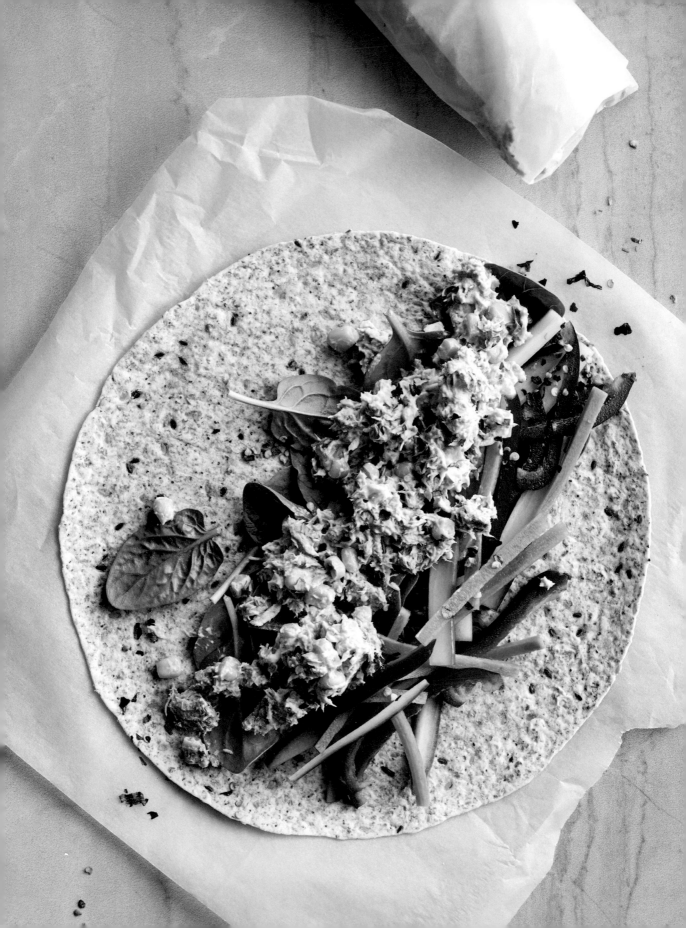

TUNA MAYO, SWEETCORN & SPINACH WRAP

PER SERVING | **339 CALS** | **31G PROTEIN** | **6G FAT** | **37G CARBS**

10 MINS

MAKES 2 WRAPS

2 white or wholegrain
   wraps
50g spinach
2 x 145g tins of tuna,
   drained
80g sweetcorn
80g low-fat mayonnaise
juice of ¹/2 a lemon
¹/4 of a cucumber
1 carrot
1 pepper (any colour)
optional: chilli flakes
salt and pepper

To serve:
2 tsp piccalilli

*Make sure the wraps
are at room temperature
or they'll rip when you
roll them.*

*This is the perfect solution for when you have food that
could soon be going out of date or some veggies or salad
that are starting to look a little sorry for themselves.
As almost any vegetable or salad item can go in a wrap
it's a great way to use up your leftovers.*

1 Place each wrap on top of a square of baking paper that's
slightly bigger. Add a line of the spinach to each wrap.

2 Mix the tuna and sweetcorn with the mayonnaise, season
and add a squeeze of lemon juice. (If you have any herbs such
as parsley lying around, add those too.)

3 Divide the tuna mixture between each wrap. Chop the
cucumber, carrot and pepper into thin sticks and add them
in lines to the wraps. I like to add some chilli flakes to mine
at this point as well.

4 Roll up the wraps inside the baking paper and seal with
tape. The wraps will keep in the fridge for up to 3 days.
I like to have mine with a side of piccalilli!

FRIDGE FORAGE VEGETABLE & LENTIL BOWLS

PER SERVING | **406** CALS | **19G** PROTEIN | **23G** FAT | **28G** CARBS

10 MINS   30 MINS

SERVES 2

200g of mixed vegetables (such as sweet potato, red pepper, butternut squash, courgette), chopped into bite-sized pieces

1/2 tsp paprika or mixed herbs

1 tbsp olive oil

2 eggs

120g Puy lentils (you can use brown rice or tinned lentils instead but remember that this will change the calories)

2 handfuls of mixed salad leaves, cooked greens or leftover raw vegetables

salt and pepper

For the dressing:

2 tbsp fat-free Greek yoghurt

1 clove of garlic, peeled and crushed

2 tbsp olive oil

juice of 1/2 a lime

This is a fantastic way to use up any leftover vegetables you have in your fridge and is packed full of nutrients! It's also super quick to whip up, which means you have no excuse to skip meal prep.

1 Preheat the oven to 220°C. Line a roasting tray with baking paper and put the vegetables on to it along with the paprika or mixed herbs, olive oil and seasoning. Mix it all together so that everything is evenly coated. Roast in the oven for 20–30 minutes, shaking the tray halfway through, until everything is cooked through and done to your liking.

2 Boil the eggs for 7 minutes and set aside to cool in a bowl of cold water, then peel and cut into quarters.

3 Mix the Greek yoghurt, garlic, olive oil and lime juice together for the dressing and season to taste.

4 Divide the roast vegetables, lentils, hard-boiled eggs, salad and any extra veg between two airtight containers. Split the dressing between two small pots and add to the meal prep containers. This will keep in the fridge for up to 3 days.

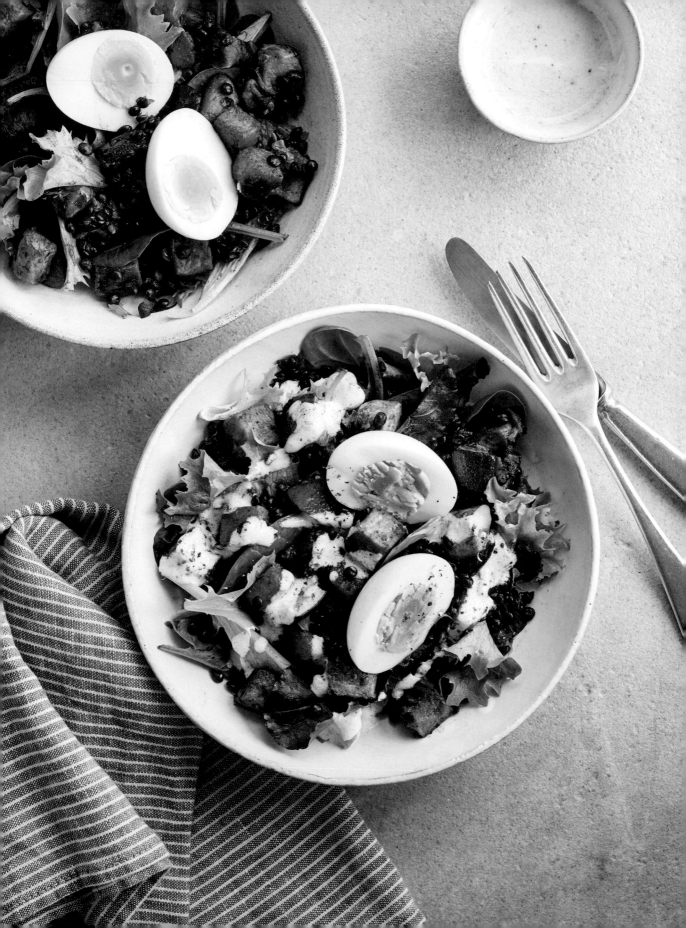

FAKE-AWAY CHICKEN FRIED RICE

PER SERVING | **463** CALS | **26G** PROTEIN | **12G** FAT | **59G** CARBS

prep 5 MINS **cook** 20 MINS **FREEZE**

SERVES 2

100g uncooked white
   or brown rice (or 200g
   if using premade)
2 tsp coconut oil
1 onion, diced
1 red pepper, diced
1 chicken breast
100g frozen peas
1 egg
3 spring onions,
   finely chopped
3 tbsp soy sauce
salt and pepper

tip

*It's best to freeze or
refrigerate rice as soon
as possible after cooking
it, once it's cooled down.
It'll keep in the fridge
for up to 1 day. When
reheating, make sure
it is steaming hot all
the way through. Do
not reheat cooked
rice more than once.*

*Did someone say Chinese takeaway? A great alternative
to a much-loved favourite, without the calories and guilt,
that can be enjoyed any day of the week.*

1 Cook the rice according to the packet instructions
or use pre-prepared rice to save time.

2 In a large pan or wok, use 1 teaspoon of coconut oil to
fry the onion and red pepper for 8–10 minutes until soft.

3 Cut the chicken into bite-sized pieces and add to the pan
along with the frozen peas and cook for 2–3 minutes. Then
crack in the egg and stir continuously until it resembles
scrambled egg: this will take 30 seconds–1 minute.

4 Add the spring onions, 1 teaspoon of coconut oil and the soy
sauce along with a good pinch of sea salt and pepper, followed
by the rice. Give it a good mix and cover. Allow to cook for
a further 5 minutes until the chicken is thoroughly cooked.

5 Divide between two airtight containers. This will keep in
the fridge for up to 1 day or in the freezer for up to 3 months.

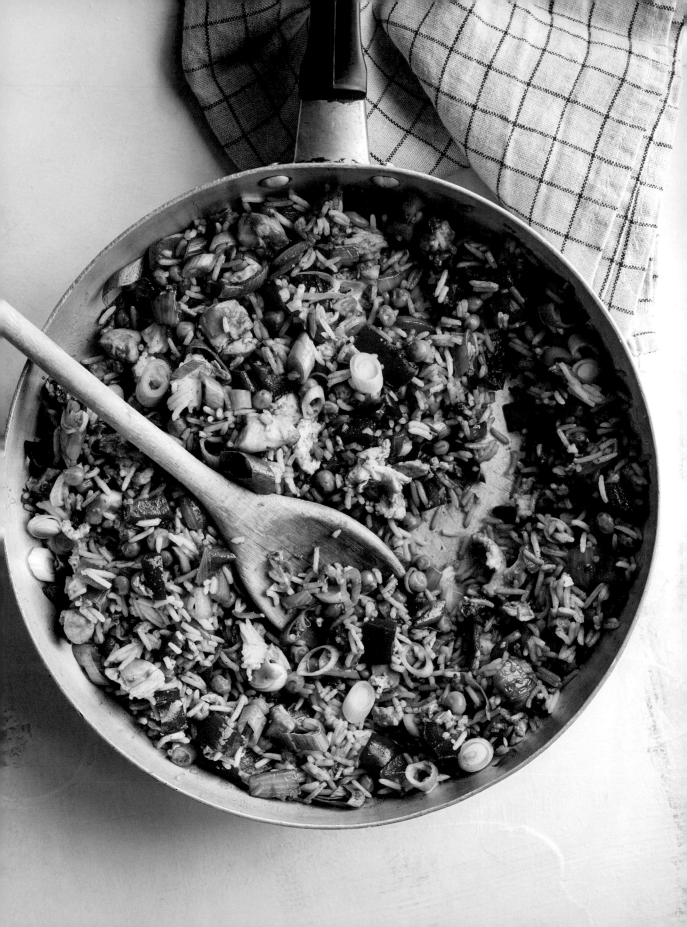

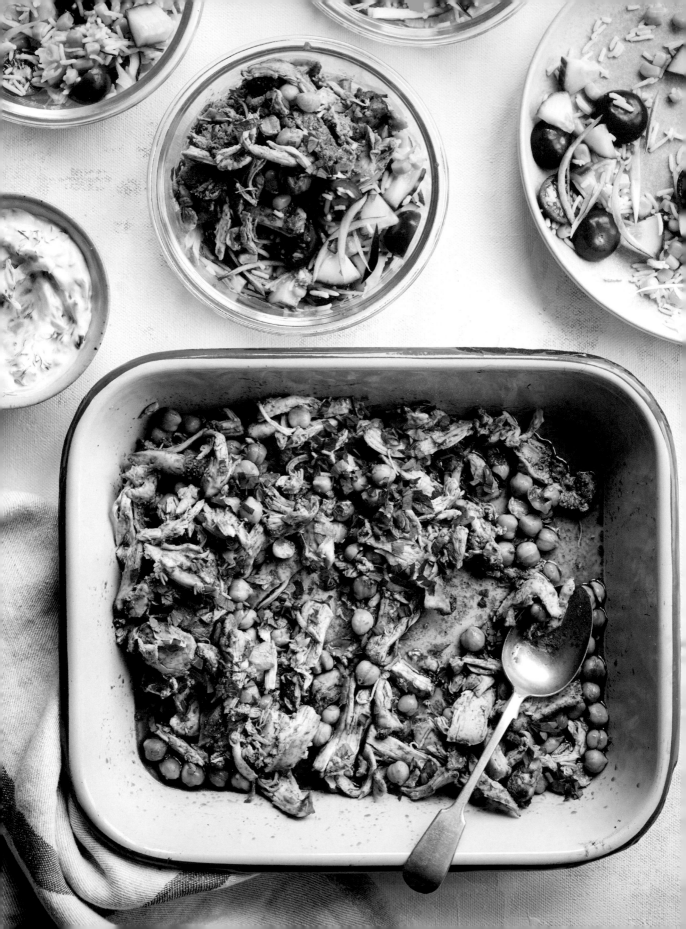

SHAWARMA CHICKEN BOWLS

PER SERVING | **495** CALS | **38G** PROTEIN | **22G** FAT | **33G** CARBS

10 MINS 30 MINS
+
MARINATING

SERVES 2

4 chicken thighs,
    skinless and boneless
2 tsp olive oil
1/2 x 400g tin of
    chickpeas, drained
100g cooked white rice
50g red onion, sliced
50g sweetcorn
100g cherry tomatoes,
    halved
100g cucumber, diced
a small handful of fresh
    parsley, chopped

*For the shawarma spice
mix (or use ready-made
mix, to taste):*
2 tsp ground cumin
2 tsp ground coriander
2 tsp paprika
1 tsp ground turmeric
1/2 tsp cayenne pepper
a pinch of ground cinnamon
1 garlic clove, crushed
salt and pepper

*Optional: for the
tzatziki sauce:*
1 garlic clove
a small handful of fresh
    dill or mint
100g low-fat Greek yoghurt
50g cucumber
1 tsp white wine vinegar

*A Middle Eastern inspired recipe that's full of flavour.
It's normally prepared with lamb but using chicken instead
keeps the all-important calorie count low, with no compromise
in flavour. The shawarma spice mix infuses the chicken
perfectly as well, making this a dish you'll keep on
returning to time and time again.*

1 Combine the ingredients for the shawarma spice mix
together in a bowl. Tip two-thirds of it into an airtight
container with the chicken thighs and olive oil, mix to make
sure the chicken is fully coated, then cover and leave to
marinate in the fridge, overnight if possible, though an
hour will also suffice. Use the remaining third of the spice
mix to coat the drained chickpeas.

2 Preheat the oven to 200°C. Remove the chicken from
the fridge and allow it to reach room temperature. Tip into
a roasting tin along with the chickpeas, cover with tin foil
and roast in the oven for 20 minutes.

3 Take the chicken out of the oven, remove the foil and
shred the meat using two forks. Return to the oven and cook
(uncovered) for 10 minutes.

4 Whilst the chicken is cooking, mix the rice, onions,
sweetcorn, cherry tomatoes and cucumber together in a
bowl, then divide between two airtight containers. Add half
the chicken and chickpeas to each container. If you're eating
straight away, sprinkle the parsley over the entire dish. It will
keep in the fridge for up to 1 day, or the chicken will keep
in the freezer for up to 3 months.

Recipe continued overleaf

5 To make the optional tzatziki sauce, finely chop the garlic and dill, then stir into the yoghurt. Grate the cucumber and squeeze the excess water out with a tea towel. Mix into the yoghurt along with the white wine vinegar and season to taste. Store in a small pot separate from the main meal (and be sure to add in the extra calories if you're using this sauce).

Top tip: You can make the chicken ahead of time if you wish. It will keep in the freezer for up to 3 months. It's best to freeze or refrigerate rice as soon as possible after cooking it, once it's cooled down. It'll keep in the fridge for up to 1 day. When reheating, make sure it is steaming hot all the way through. Do not reheat cooked rice more than once.

HOT PEPPERED HONEY-GLAZED SALMON

PER SERVING | **439** CALS | **31G** PROTEIN | **16G** FAT | **41G** CARBS

5 MINS   25 MINS
+
MARINATING

SERVES 2

2 salmon fillets
1 tsp olive oil
150g mangetout
100g couscous
1 vegetable stock cube

For the marinade:
1 tsp pink peppercorns
1 tsp black peppercorns
a pinch of sea salt
1/4 tsp chilli powder
1 tbsp olive oil
2 cloves of garlic, peeled
   and finely chopped
2 tbsp chopped fresh dill
10g honey
juice of 1/2 a lemon

You can cook the salmon as per the method opposite and it will keep in the freezer for up to 3 months. When you reheat it, all you'll have to do is cook the couscous and mangetout to go with it.

This recipe is a seafood favourite of Charlotte's. She loves salmon, so when I meal prep this I have to be quick to eat one or she'll eat both! The honey-glaze marinade takes this recipe to a whole new level.

1 In a bowl, grind the peppercorns and sea salt together and mix in the chilli powder. Mix the olive oil, the spice seasoning, garlic, dill, honey and lemon juice together in an airtight container, then add the fish and make sure it's fully coated with the mixture. For best results, cover and place in the fridge overnight to marinate; however, 2–3 hours will do if you're pushed for time.

2 Preheat the oven to 200°C. Heat the olive oil in a frying pan over a high heat. Fry the salmon fillets skin side down for 2–3 minutes until crispy. Then wrap them in tin foil to form a parcel and bake in the oven for 15–20 minutes until fully cooked.

3 Whilst the fish is cooking, steam the mangetout for 1–2 minutes and divide them between two airtight containers.

4 Combine the couscous with the vegetable stock cube and cook according to the packet instructions, then add it to the meal prep containers.

5 Top each meal prep container with a slice of cooked fish and add a slice of lemon to each tub. Sprinkle any leftover dill you may have. This meal will keep in the fridge for up to 3 days.

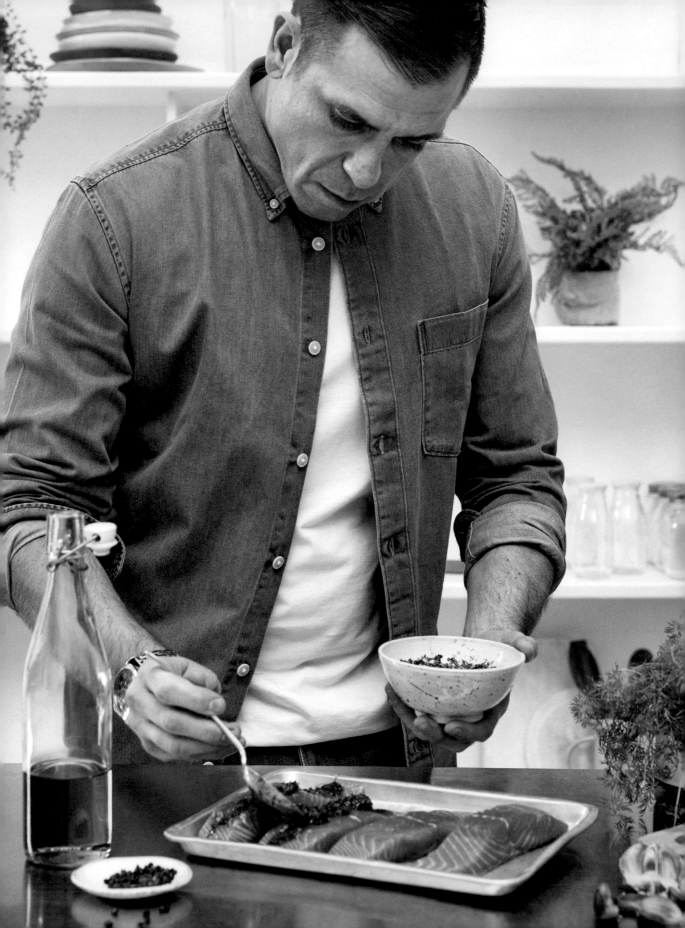

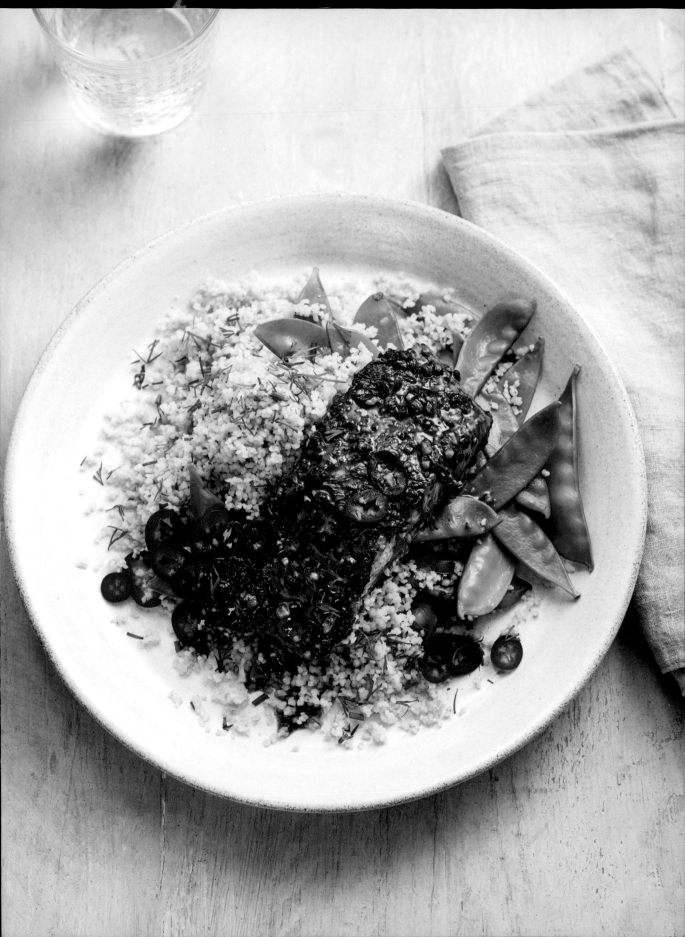

GARLIC CHICKEN & KALE SPAGHETTI

PER SERVING | **492** CALS | **40G** PROTEIN | **17G** FAT | **40G** CARBS

10 MINS   20 MINS   FREEZE

SERVES 2

2 chicken breasts (about 250g)
1/2 tsp garlic powder
1/2 tsp onion salt
1 tbsp olive oil
120g wholegrain spaghetti
4 cloves of garlic, peeled
10g unsalted butter
optional: 100g mushrooms,
   sliced
60g kale
20g Parmesan cheese, grated
a small handful of fresh
   flat-leaf parsley, chopped
salt and pepper

It's no secret that the water from cooked pasta is like an extra ingredient in itself. The pasta releases starch when cooked, which means that the water becomes a great thickener for sauces, which will change your pasta dishes from average to silky smooth! So please save a cupful once you've cooked your pasta to add to the sauce – you won't regret it.

A quick and simple chicken pasta dish that is perfect to eat at work or on the go. And you can always swap out the kale for any other greens you might have in the fridge.

1 Preheat the oven to 200°C. Put the chicken breasts between two sheets of baking paper or clingfilm and bash with a rolling pin until they are the same thickness all over (this ensures even cooking). Season them with salt and pepper, garlic powder and onion salt.

2 Heat the olive oil in a frying pan over a medium to high heat. Fry the chicken for 1 minute on either side to seal. Then wrap the chicken in foil and cook in the oven for 20 minutes.

3 Bring a large pan of generously salted water to the boil. Add the spaghetti and cook for 1 minute less than the packet instructions so it's al dente. Reserve 1 cup of pasta water and then drain.

4 Finely chop the garlic cloves. Melt the butter in a saucepan over a low heat then add the garlic and cook for 1–2 minutes whilst stirring continuously. If you're using mushrooms, sauté them with the garlic – it will take 4–5 minutes.

5 Steam the kale for 1–2 minutes (you can do this in a steamer or in the microwave).

6 Mix the spaghetti into the garlic sauce and add 2–3 tablespoons of the pasta water to loosen it up. Then cut the cooked chicken into bite-sized pieces and add it to the pasta along with the kale. Divide between two airtight containers and sprinkle with the Parmesan cheese and parsley. This will keep in the fridge for up to 3 days.

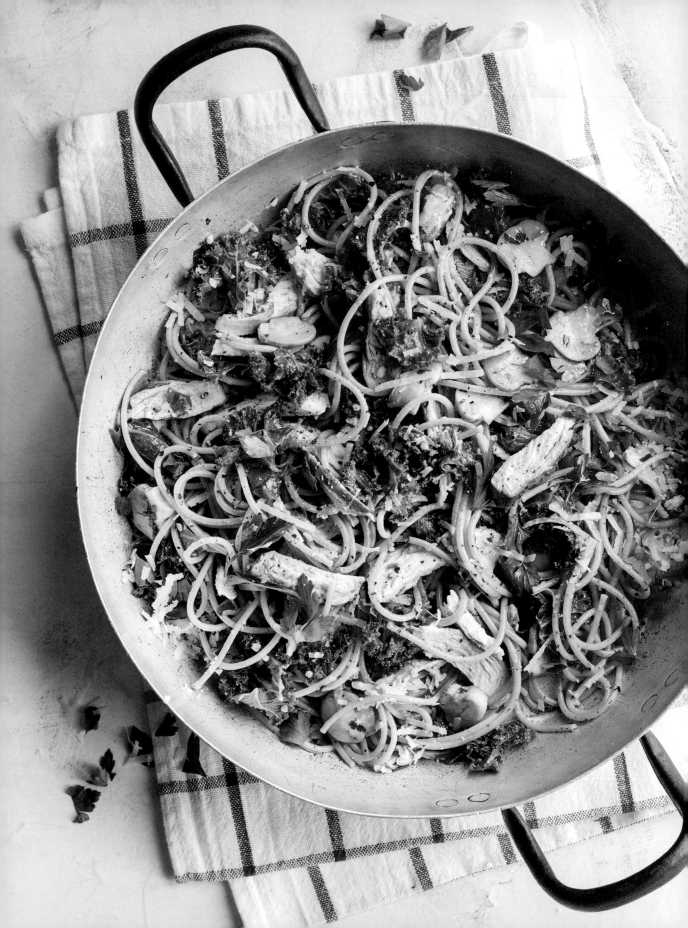

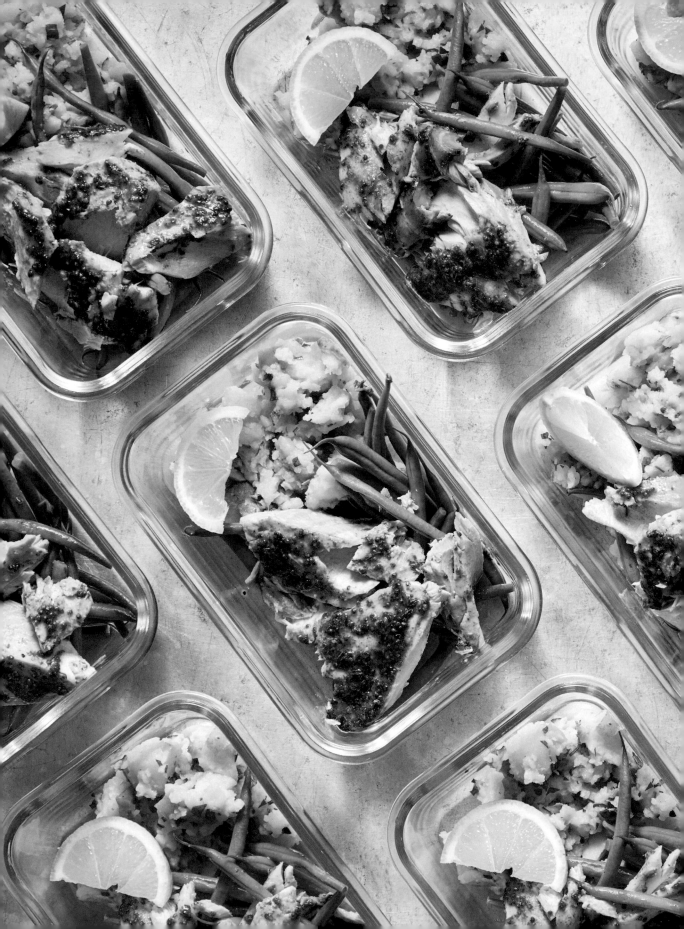

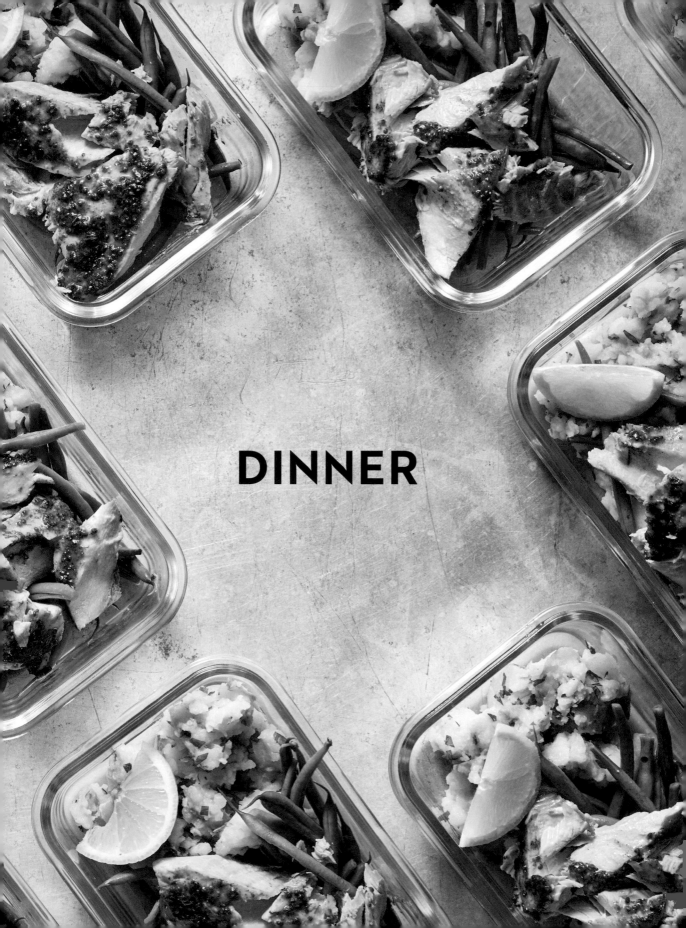

DINNER

RED LENTIL BURGERS

PER SERVING IF BAKING | 251 CALS | 12G PROTEIN | 7G FAT | 33G CARBS
PER SERVING IF FRYING | 278 CALS | 12G PROTEIN | 10G FAT | 33G CARBS
WITH A BURGER BUN | ADD 159 CALS | 6G PROTEIN | 1G FAT | 30 CARBS

10 MIN   25 MINS   40 MINS
IF FRIED   IF BAKED

SERVES 2

50g red lentils
1 bay leaf
1/2 tbsp olive oil (you'll need
   an extra 1/2 tbsp if you're
   frying the burger)
1/2 a carrot, finely diced
1/2 an onion, finely chopped
2 rashers of bacon, diced
30g rolled oats
20g breadcrumbs
1 tsp soy sauce
a handful of fresh
   coriander, roughly
   chopped
salt and pepper

To serve:
chilli jam
mixed leaf salad
cherry tomatoes,
   sliced in half
optional: 2 burger buns

*Check out the world
food aisle in your local
supermarket where red
lentils tend to be sold in
larger quantities and at a
lower price. If you want the
burgers to be vegetarian,
leave out the bacon.*

*Red lentils are a staple in Frank's house and I've eaten
a lot of them! These lentils are packed with protein and are
an extremely cheap meal prep option. The joy of this recipe
is that you can have the red lentil burgers with or without
a bun, and you can fry or bake them as well.*

1 Bring 250ml of water to the boil, then add the red lentils
and bay leaf. Gently simmer the lentils for 15–20 minutes,
stirring occasionally to stop them sticking, until tender.
Drain any excess water and remove the bay leaf.

2 Whilst the lentils are cooking, heat half a tablespoon
of olive oil in a frying pan over a medium heat and add the
carrot, onion and bacon. Fry them for 8–10 minutes, stirring
occasionally, until they're soft.

3 Blitz the oats in a food processor until they've turned into
a powder. Mix the oat flour and breadcrumbs with the cooked
ingredients along with the soy sauce and chopped coriander.
Shape the mixture into two burgers.

4 If you're frying, heat half a tablespoon of olive oil in a frying
pan over a medium heat and cook the burgers for 2 minutes
on either side until golden brown. If you're baking, preheat the
oven to 200°C and cook the burgers for 20 minutes, turning
them over halfway.

5 They will keep in the fridge for up to 3 days or in the freezer
for up to 3 months. If you're eating them straight away, top
them with some chilli jam, put them in a burger bun (if using)
and serve with a mixed leaf salad and cherry tomatoes.

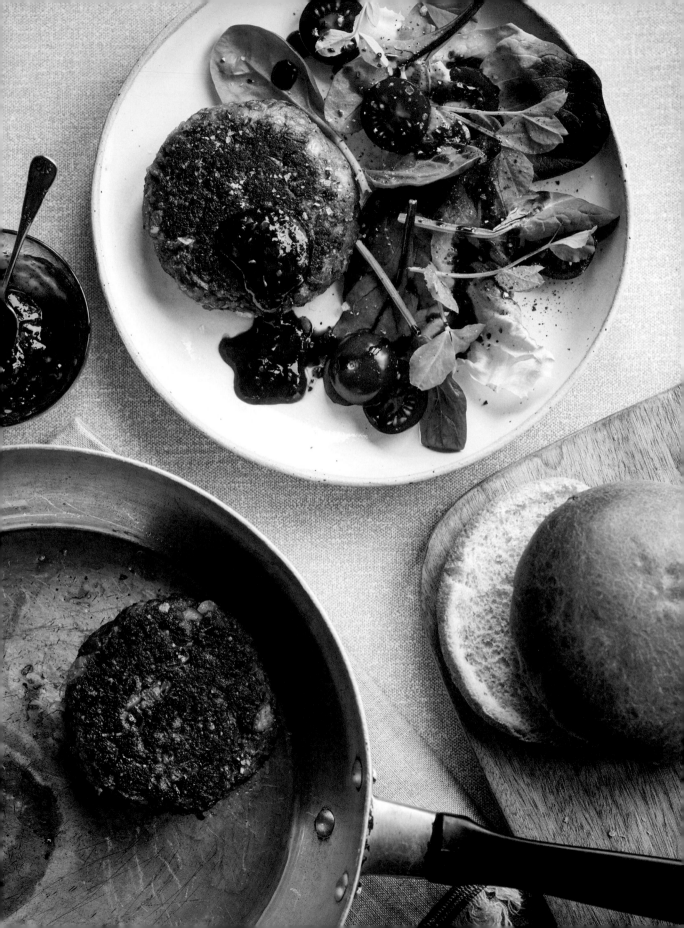

PERI PERI CHICKEN BURGERS

PER SERVING | **449** CALS | **39G** PROTEIN | **18G** FAT | **32G** CARBS

10 MINS   25 MINS

SERVES 2

2 chicken breasts
   (about 300g in total)
1 tbsp rapeseed oil
2 brioche buns
1 large beef tomato, sliced
1/2 a gem lettuce, leaves
   separated
50g red onion, sliced
30g light mayonnaise

**For the peri peri seasoning
(or use a ready-made mix,
to taste):**
2 tsp paprika
1 tsp onion powder
1 tsp garlic powder
1 tsp ground cardamom
1/2 tsp ground ginger
1/4 tsp caster sugar
1 tsp dried oregano
1/2 tsp cayenne pepper
salt and pepper

*Make sure you store the
chicken breast, salad and
bun separately if using for
meal prep, and construct
the burger when you're
ready to eat. If you want a
lighter dinner, leave out the
bun and have the chicken
with a salad or some rice.
The chicken will keep in the
freezer for up to 3 months.*

*Do you like spice and heat? Then these peri peri chicken
burgers are ideal. Try adding a teaspoon of extra hot chilli
powder to the seasoning for that extra burn!*

1 Put the chicken breasts between two sheets of baking
paper or clingfilm and bash with a rolling pin until they are
the same thickness all over (this ensures even cooking).
Then place the chicken in an airtight container or a ziplock
food bag with half a tablespoon of the rapeseed oil and add
the peri peri seasoning. Mix so that the chicken is completely
covered. Leave to marinate overnight in the fridge if you
can, but don't worry, even 10 minutes will work well.

2 Preheat the oven to 200°C. Take the chicken out of
the fridge 10 minutes before you plan on cooking it. Heat the
remainder of the oil in a frying pan over a medium-high heat
and fry the chicken for 1 minute on each side to seal it.

3 Put the chicken breasts into a roasting tin and roast in the
oven for 20 minutes until the juices run clear when you poke
the meat with a knife.

4 Construct your burger: place the peri peri chicken on top
of a brioche bun base, then add a couple of slices of beef
tomato, some lettuce leaves, red onion and mayonnaise. Enjoy!
The chicken will keep in the fridge for up to 3 days.

CHICKPEA BURGERS

PER SERVING | **490** CALS | **17G** PROTEIN | **16G** FAT | **65G** CARBS

30 MINS 10 MINS

SERVES 2

1 x 400g tin of
   chickpeas, drained
1 tbsp flour
juice of 1 lemon
1/2 tsp ground cumin
1/2 tsp ground coriander
1/2 tsp paprika
1/2 tsp ground turmeric
1/2 tsp garlic powder
1/2 tsp onion granules
a small handful of
   fresh coriander,
   roughly chopped
40g breadcrumbs
1 tbsp olive oil
2 brioche buns, beetroot
   ones if you can find them
1 beef tomato, sliced
1 mini gem lettuce,
   leaves separated
50g red onion, sliced
light mayonnaise
salt and pepper

*Remember to store
the burger and the bun
separately if using for
meal prep. You can make
the burgers ahead if you
wish and they will keep
in the freezer for up
to 3 months.*

*Chickpeas make an excellent alternative to meat and they're
high in protein and fibre. Once you have tried these burgers,
I guarantee you'll make them again and again.*

1 Put the chickpeas, flour, lemon juice, cumin, coriander, paprika,
turmeric, garlic powder, onion granules, chopped coriander
and salt and pepper into a food processor and blend until
smooth. (This can be done by hand using a potato masher
if you don't have a food processor.)

2 Mix in half the breadcrumbs and shape the mixture into
two burgers, then coat in the remaining breadcrumbs. Chill
in the fridge for 20 minutes.

3 Heat the olive oil in a frying pan over a medium to low heat
and fry the burgers for 4–5 minutes on each side until golden
brown (reduce the heat if they look like they're getting too
much colour).

4 The burgers will keep in the fridge for up to 3 days or
in the freezer for up to 3 months. To construct your burger,
place the chickpea burger on top of a brioche bun base,
then add a couple of slices of beef tomato, some lettuce
leaves, sliced red onion and light mayonnaise. Enjoy!

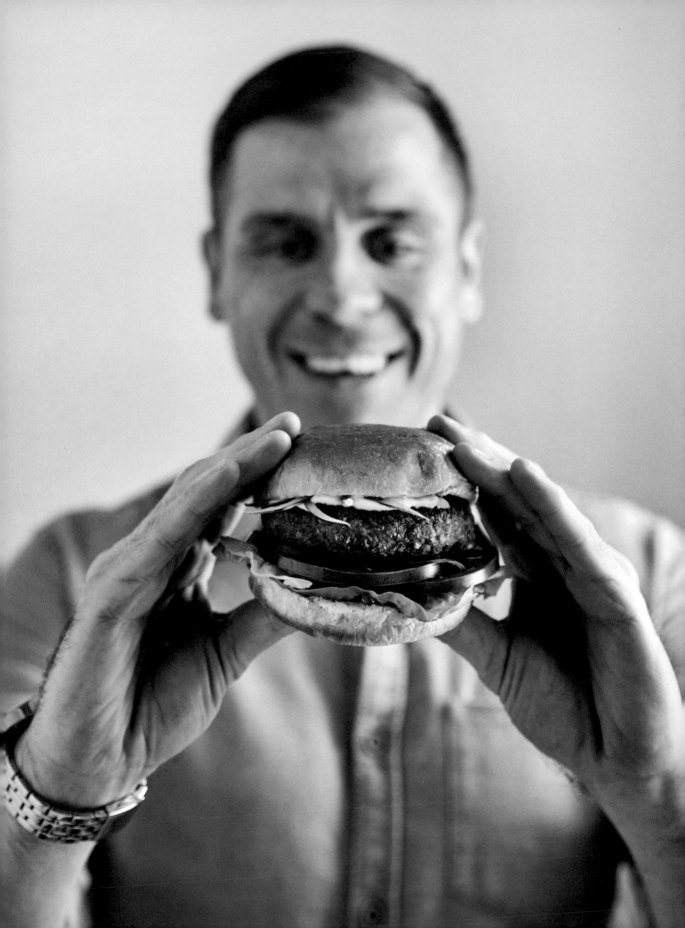

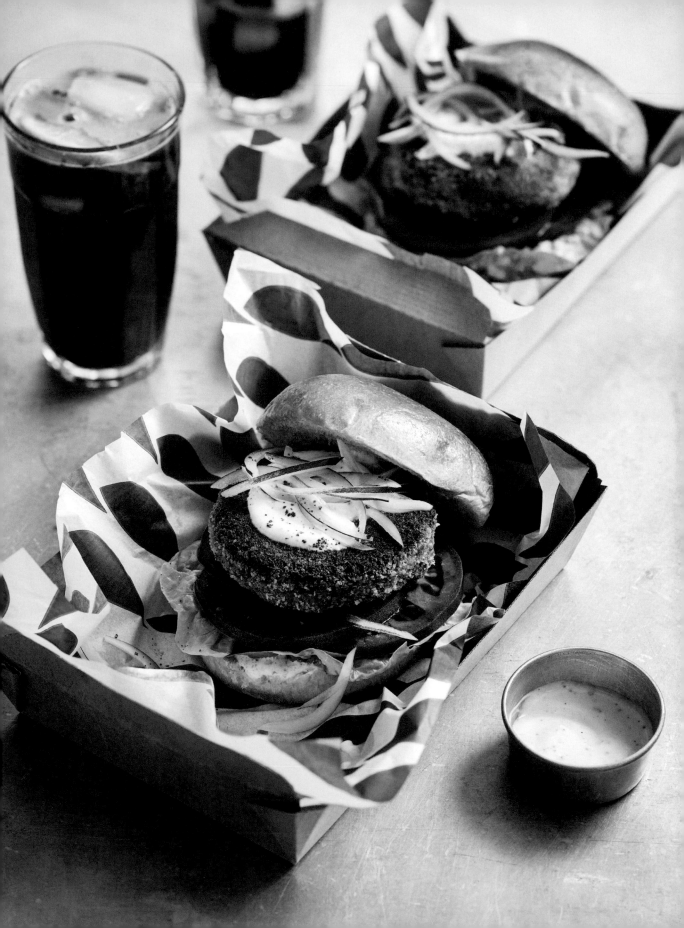

CHARLOTTE'S LASAGNE

PER SERVING | **478** CALS | **35G** PROTEIN | **14G** FAT | **50G** CARBS

prep **10 MINS** cook **65 MINS** **FREEZE**

SERVES 4

low-cal spray oil
1 onion, diced
2 cloves of garlic,
    peeled and crushed
400g 5% fat lean
    beef mince
400g passata
1 tbsp Worcestershire
    sauce
a handful of fresh basil
    leaves, roughly chopped
25g unsalted butter
15g plain flour
300ml semi-skimmed milk
30g Parmesan cheese,
    coarsely grated
200g fresh egg lasagne
    sheets
1/2 tsp dried oregano
optional: 80g mixed
    salad leaves
salt and pepper

I love it when Charlotte makes this lasagne as it's very filling and tasty. It's great to make on your own or as a couple for that extra bonding time. Sometimes two cooks are better than one in the kitchen!

1 To make the ragù, heat a large frying pan over a medium heat and spray with low-cal oil. Fry the onion and garlic for 8–10 minutes until softened.

2 Add the mince and continue to fry for 7–10 minutes until the meat is fully browned. Stir in the passata, Worcestershire sauce and 100ml of water, bring to the boil, then reduce to a simmer for 15 minutes or until the liquid has reduced. Sprinkle with the chopped basil and season.

3 To make the béchamel sauce, melt the butter in a small saucepan over a low heat and add the plain flour, whisking for 1–2 minutes until combined. Gradually whisk in the milk very slowly until you have a glossy sauce, then add 15g of the Parmesan cheese, whisking constantly until the sauce thickens.

4 Preheat the oven to 200°C. In an ovenproof baking dish, start with a base layer of the ragù, followed by a layer of fresh lasagne sheets and then a layer of the white béchamel sauce. Repeat this step twice.

5 Lastly, sprinkle the remaining Parmesan cheese and the dried oregano all over the top and bake in the centre of the oven for 30–40 minutes, until the lasagne is piping hot and the cheese is golden and bubbling. Allow to cool completely before slicing into four portions.

6 Divide the mixed salad leaves, if using, between four airtight containers and top with a slice of lasagne – but don't include the salad leaves if you intend to freeze the lasagne. It will keep in the fridge for up to 3 days or in the freezer for up to 3 months.

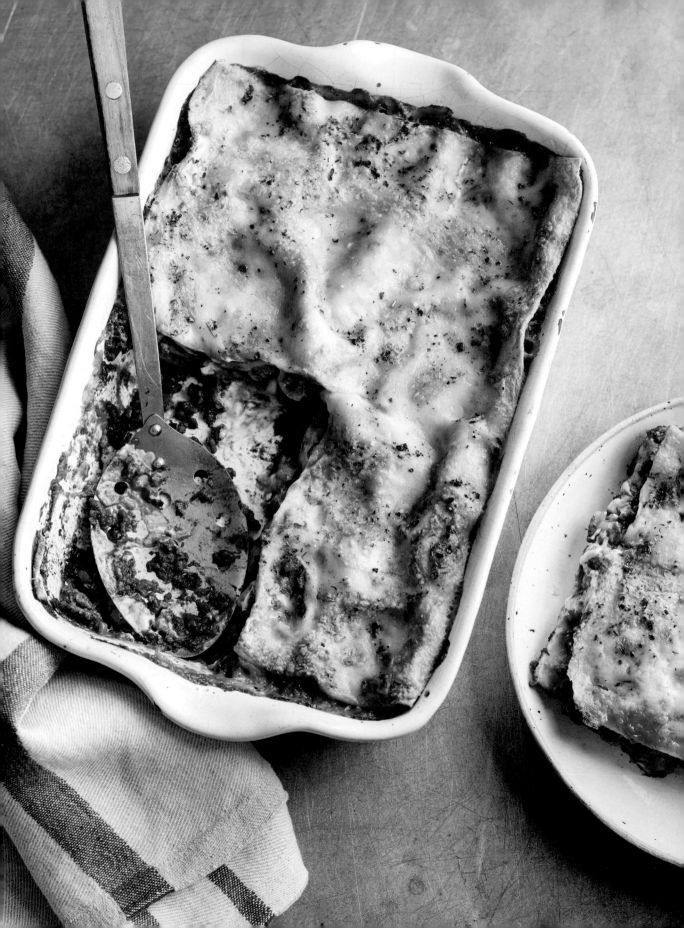

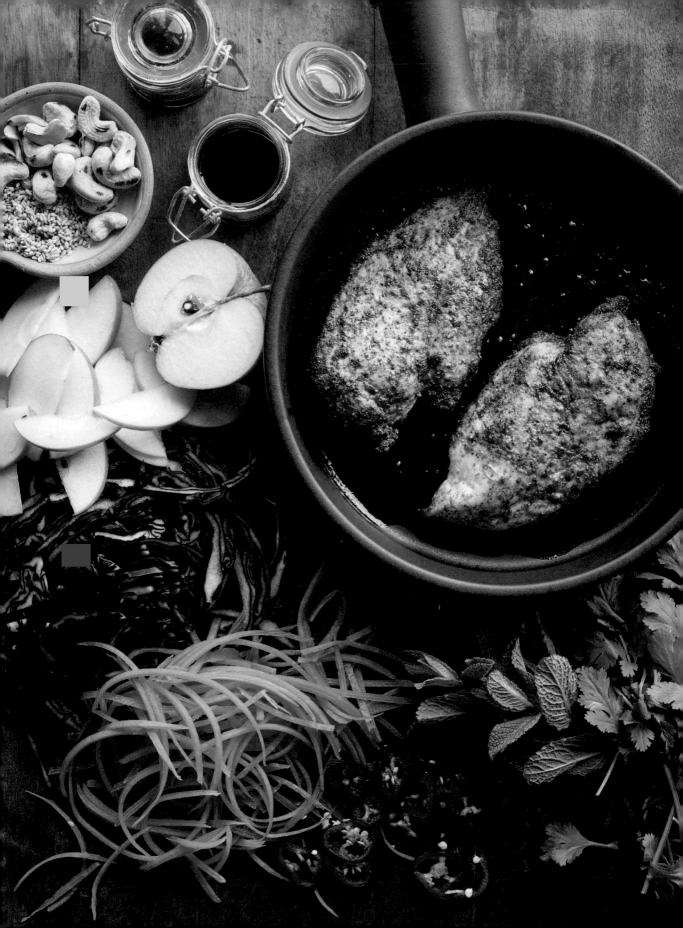

THAI CHICKEN WITH ASIAN-STYLE SLAW

PER SERVING | **477** CALS | **35G** PROTEIN | **30G** FAT | **14G** CARBS

10 MINS   25 MINS

SERVES 2

2 chicken breasts
1 tbsp olive oil

For the Thai spice mix (or use a ready-made mix, to taste):
1/2 tsp ground cumin
1 tbsp lemon pepper
1/2 tsp chilli powder
1/2 tsp garlic powder
1 tsp ground ginger
1/2 tsp onion powder
salt and pepper

For the slaw:
100g red or green cabbage
1/2 a green apple
1 carrot
30g roasted peanuts
   or cashew nuts
1 tbsp toasted sesame seeds
a small handful of fresh
   mint and coriander
   leaves, chopped
optional: 1 red chilli,
   finely chopped

For the dressing:
2 tsp sesame oil
2 tbsp soy sauce
juice of 1/2 a lemon
1 tbsp extra-virgin olive oil

You can make the chicken ahead of time if you wish. It will keep in the freezer for up to 3 months.

The combination of fresh ingredients and vibrant colours in this dish makes this meal prep heaven, and the flavours are amazing. Whilst normal coleslaw is delicious, this Thai one is even tastier and healthier!

1 Put the chicken breasts between two sheets of baking paper or clingfilm and bash with a rolling pin until they are the same thickness all over (this ensures even cooking). Then put the chicken into an airtight container along with half a tablespoon of the olive oil and the spice mix. Mix everything together, making sure that the chicken is fully coated. Leave to marinate in the fridge overnight if possible, or for at least an hour before cooking.

2 To make the slaw, thinly slice the cabbage, apple and carrot. Put them in a bowl and mix in the nuts, toasted seeds, herbs and red chilli, if using. Mix all the ingredients for the dressing together.

3 To cook the chicken, preheat the oven to 180°C. Heat the remaining olive oil in a frying pan over a high heat and fry the chicken for 1–2 minutes on each side until golden brown. Place the chicken in a roasting tin and roast in the oven for 20–25 minutes until fully cooked.

4 If it's for meal prep, divide the slaw between two airtight containers and top with the chicken. Split the dressing between two little pots and add one to each container. This will keep in the fridge for up to 3 days. When you're ready to eat, pour the dressing over the slaw and serve with the chicken.

STUFFED SWEET POTATOES WITH BUFFALO SAUCE

PER SERVING | **431 CALS** | **29G PROTEIN** | **25G FAT** | **21G CARBS**

10 MINS **6.5 HOURS** **FREEZE**

SERVES 4

50g butter, cubed
100ml hot sauce
3 tbsp coconut oil
1/2 tsp garlic powder
1/2 tsp cayenne pepper
3 chicken breasts
   (500g in total)
4 small sweet potatoes
salt and pepper

To serve:
ranch dressing
a small handful of fresh
   chives, chopped

Sweet potatoes are an absolute meal prep king favourite. This little red potato is so versatile, as not only is it packed full of nutrients and flavour but it goes with almost anything. Stuffed with chicken and a hot buffalo sauce, this meal prep recipe will certainly get those taste buds going.

1 Heat a small saucepan over a medium-high heat and put in the butter, hot sauce, coconut oil, garlic powder and cayenne pepper. Stir until the butter is melted and everything is combined into a smooth sauce.

2 Pour the sauce into a slow cooker, add the chicken breasts and cook for 4–6 hours on low, until the chicken is tender.

3 Meanwhile, roast the sweet potatoes. Preheat the oven to 220°C and line a baking tray with foil. Prick the potatoes all over with a fork and roast them in the oven for 40–50 minutes until soft.

4 Shred the chicken in the slow cooker with a fork, then re-cover it and leave it to cook for a further 30 minutes. Season to taste.

5 If it's for meal prep, place a sweet potato in each of four airtight containers and divide the chicken equally between them. They will keep in the fridge for up to 3 days or in the freezer for up to 3 months. If you're eating right away, divide the chicken equally between the sweet potatoes and drizzle with ranch dressing (taking into account the extra calories), if desired, then top with chives.

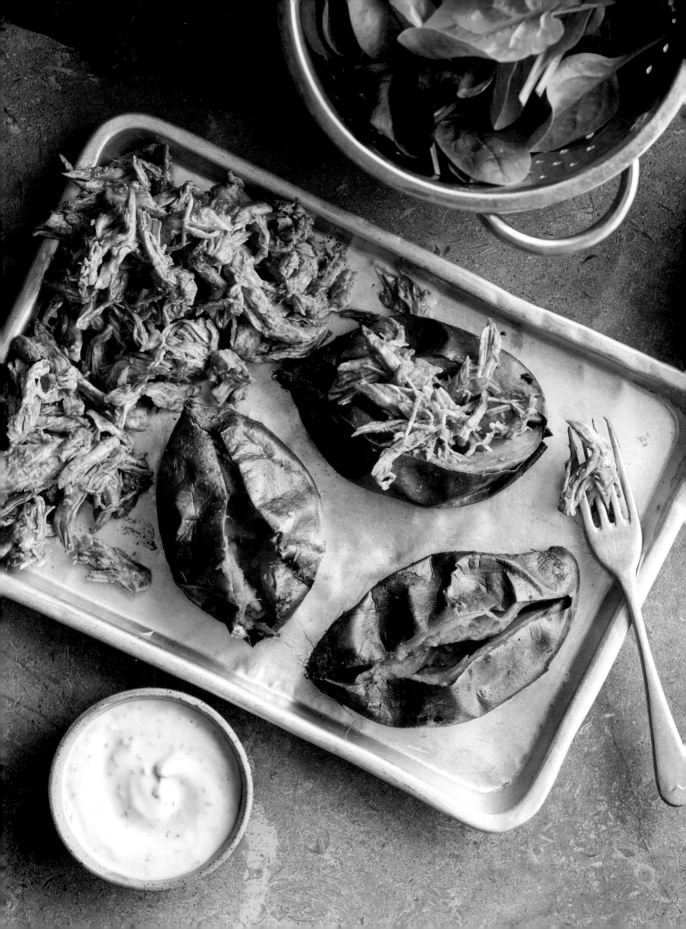

LANCASHIRE HOT POT & PICKLED RED CABBAGE

PER SERVING | 485 CALS | 26G PROTEIN | 18G FAT | 49G CARBS

prep 20 MINS **cook** 1 HOUR 40 MINS **FREEZE**

SERVES 2

200g lean lamb meat
(all excess fat trimmed),
cut into bite-sized pieces
10g flour
2 tsp olive oil
1 onion, sliced
2 tbsp Worcestershire sauce
1 vegetable stock cube
1 tbsp tomato purée
100g carrot, peeled and sliced
100g leeks, sliced
bouquet garni
300g potatoes, peeled and
thinly sliced
optional: 3 sprigs of thyme,
leaves picked
salt and pepper

For the pickled red cabbage:
200g red cabbage
300ml white wine vinegar
(enough to cover
the cabbage)

*If freezing, don't include
the pickled red cabbage.*

Being from Lancashire, I thought it only right to include a locally inspired family favourite. Traditionally enjoyed on Bonfire Night, this recipe brings back memories of my childhood. Pickled red cabbage is a great accompaniment to the hot pot. It's incredibly easy to make, will keep for up to a month in the fridge and is much cheaper than shop-bought versions too.

1 Pickle the cabbage the night before. Thinly slice the cabbage and put it in a glass jar along with a large pinch of salt and the white wine vinegar (enough to cover the cabbage). Mix thoroughly, seal and leave overnight in the fridge. It will keep in the fridge for up to a month.

2 Preheat the oven to 170°C. In a bowl, mix the lamb and flour together so the lamb is fully coated. Heat 1 teaspoon of the olive oil in a saucepan over a medium heat, add the lamb and brown for 3–4 minutes. Set aside.

3 Fry the sliced onion in the same pan for 8 minutes, until starting to brown, then stir in the Worcestershire sauce. Dissolve the vegetable stock cube in 200ml of boiling water and pour into the pan.

4 Add the lamb, tomato purée, carrot and leek, then season to taste and simmer for 2–3 minutes. Divide the mixture between two individual ramekins or put it all in one small oven dish.

5 Make a well in the centre of the mixture and pop in the bouquet garni (split it into multiple smaller ones if you're using individual ramekins).

6 Arrange the sliced potatoes on top of the meat, so that they're overlapping slightly, and brush with the remaining teaspoon of olive oil. Sprinkle with thyme leaves, if using, and season. Cover with tin foil and place in the oven for around 1 hour until the potatoes are tender. To brown, remove the tin foil and place the hot pot under the grill for 5–7 minutes or turn the oven up to 200°C.

7 Divide the hot pot between two airtight containers. It will keep in the fridge for up to 3 days or in the freezer for up to 3 months. Serve with the pickled cabbage.

COMFORTING COTTAGE PIE

PER SERVING | **467** CALS | **39G** PROTEIN | **17G** FAT | **36G** CARBS

20 MINS

1 HOUR
25 MINS

FREEZE

SERVES 2

1 tbsp olive oil
250g 5% fat lean
    beef mince
1 carrot
1 onion
1 stick of celery
1 clove of garlic, peeled
    and crushed
1 x 400g tin of plum
    tomatoes, drained
1/2 a beef stock cube
1 sprig of thyme
50g frozen peas
1/2 tbsp tomato purée
1 tbsp Worcestershire
    sauce
200g sweet potatoes
20ml semi-skimmed milk
40g low-fat Cheddar
    cheese, grated
salt and pepper

Who doesn't love cottage pie? This succulent and healthy oven-baked classic is packed with delicious vegetables, lean mince and a rich meaty sauce. Delicious!

1 Put half a tablespoon of the olive oil into a saucepan over a medium heat and brown the mince for 7–10 minutes, adding the mince a bit at a time so it browns evenly. Then remove from the pan and set to one side.

2 Add the remaining olive oil to the pan and turn down the heat to low. Dice the carrot, onion and celery finely. Add to the pan along with the garlic and fry for 10–15 minutes, stirring occasionally, until soft. Add the plum tomatoes and press them down with the back of a spoon to break them up. Crumble in the stock cube and add the thyme.

3 Tip the browned mince into the saucepan, then add the frozen peas, the tomato purée, the Worcestershire sauce and 150ml water. Mix well and season to taste. Bring to the boil, then reduce to a simmer and cook for 30 minutes.

4 Preheat the oven to 200°C. Whilst the filling is cooking, make the sweet potato mash. Peel and cube the potatoes, then boil in a saucepan in salted water for 10–15 minutes until tender. Drain and return the potatoes to the heat for 20–30 seconds, stirring continually to allow any excess moisture to evaporate. Stir in the milk and mash, then season to taste.

5 Once the meat mixture is ready, pour it into an ovenproof dish. Spoon over the mashed potato and spread it evenly over the meaty base. Sprinkle over the Cheddar cheese, put into the oven and cook for 30 minutes until golden brown.

6 When the pie has cooled, divide between two airtight containers. It will keep in the fridge for up to 3 days or in the freezer for up to 3 months.

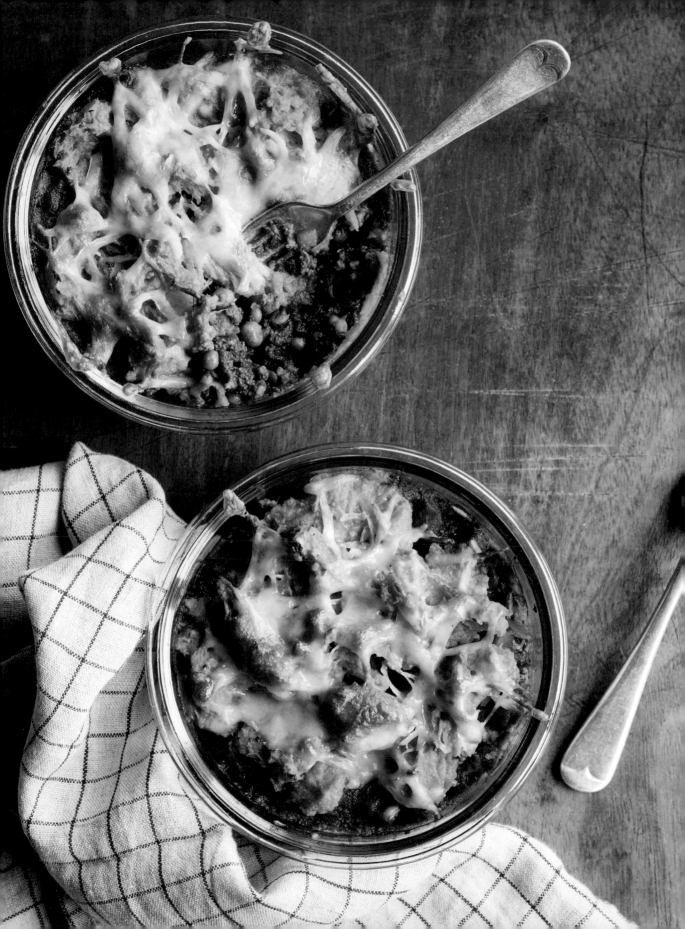

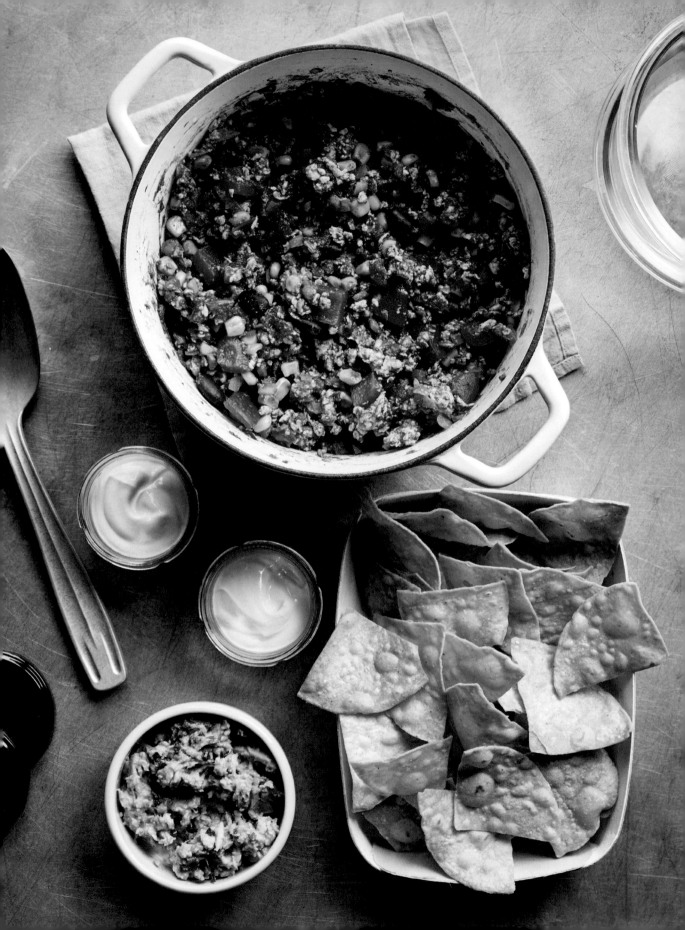

TURKEY CHILLI CON CARNE

PER SERVING | **476** CALS | **58G** PROTEIN | **20G** FAT | **33G** CARBS

10 MINS **1 HOUR** **FREEZE**

SERVES 2

1 tbsp olive oil
1 onion, finely diced
1 clove of garlic, peeled
   and crushed
1 red pepper, diced
300g lean turkey mince
1/2 tsp chilli powder
1 tsp ground cumin
1/2 tsp dried oregano
1/4 tsp cayenne pepper
1/4 tsp salt
1/2 tsp caster sugar
1 x 400g tin of chopped
   tomatoes
1/2 x 400g tin of kidney
   beans, drained and rinsed
100g sweetcorn
1 chicken stock cube
salt and pepper

To serve:
tortilla chips
guacamole
sour cream

This turkey chilli con carne is a great alternative to the usual minced-beef version. Why not try a mix of turkey and pork for an even meatier flavour?

1 Heat the olive oil in a frying pan over a medium heat and fry the onion, garlic and red pepper for 8–10 minutes until softened. Add the turkey mince to the pan and cook for 5–7 minutes before adding the chilli powder, cumin, oregano, cayenne pepper and salt.

2 Stir in the sugar, chopped tomatoes, kidney beans and sweetcorn, crumble in the chicken stock cube and add 100ml water. Bring to the boil and reduce to a simmer for 35–40 minutes until the sauce starts to thicken. Season to taste.

3 Divide between two airtight containers. The chilli will keep in the fridge for up to 3 days or in the freezer for up to 3 months. Serve with tortilla chips, guacamole and sour cream if you like (remembering to count the additional calories).

FISHERMAN'S PIE

PER SERVING | **486** CALS | **42G** PROTEIN | **18G** FAT | **35G** CARBS

10 MINS   **55 MINS**   **FREEZE**

SERVES 2

200g potatoes
100g cod
100g smoked haddock
100g salmon
200ml semi-skimmed milk
1 bay leaf
20g unsalted butter
10g plain flour
a small handful of fresh dill,
   finely chopped
20g low-fat Cheddar
   cheese
a handful of fresh parsley,
   chopped
150g frozen peas
salt and pepper

This fish pie is perfect for the whole family. Not only do adults love it but toddlers go mad for it as well. It's incredibly simple to make, especially as supermarkets sell pre-cut fish mixtures for pies and stews. You can also make it ahead of time and it reheats fantastically. A great family favourite!

1 Peel the potatoes, chop into medium-sized chunks, then cook in boiling salted water for 15–20 minutes until tender. Mash and set aside.

2 Chop the fish into bite-sized pieces. Put the milk into a saucepan and bring gently to the boil. Once it's simmering, add the fish and the bay leaf and season. Simmer for 10 minutes until the fish is cooked. Drain the milk into a jug, remove the bay leaf and set the fish aside in a bowl.

3 Preheat the oven to 200°C. Melt the butter in a small saucepan over a low heat and add in the plain flour, whisking for 1–2 minutes until combined. Gradually whisk in the fishy milk very slowly until you have a glossy sauce. Stir in the fish and the chopped dill, then season to taste.

4 Pour the fish mixture into an ovenproof dish. Top with the mashed potato, spreading it evenly all over the base. Sprinkle with the cheese and bake in the oven for 25 minutes until golden brown on top. Leave to cool and sprinkle with the chopped parsley.

5 Whilst the pie is baking, cook the frozen peas according to the packet instructions. Drain and divide between two airtight containers, then top with the cooled pie. It will keep in the fridge for up to 3 days or in the freezer for up to 3 months.

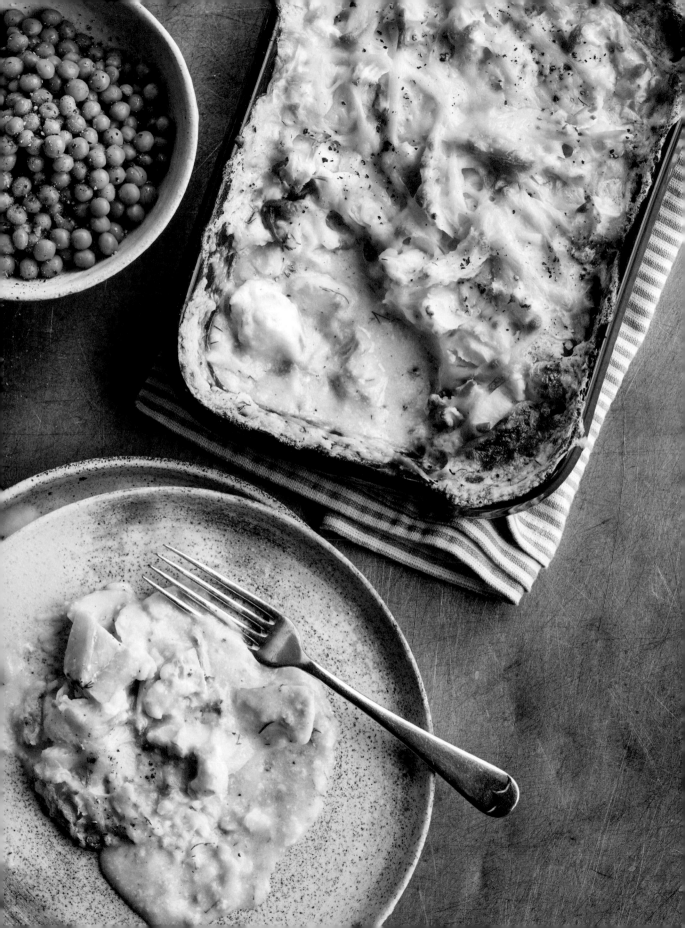

FULLY LOADED DIRTY FRIES

PER SERVING | **482** CALS | **31G** PROTEIN | **10G** FAT | **64G** CARBS

15 MINS 35 MINS FREEZE

SERVES 2

650g white potatoes
low-cal spray oil
½ a red pepper
½ a green pepper
1 tbsp vegetable oil
150g 5% fat lean beef mince
40g low-fat Cheddar
   cheese, grated
optional: 1 spring onion,
   finely sliced
optional: sweety drop
   red peppers
optional: a drizzle of
   sriracha sauce

For the spice mix:
½ tsp Chinese
   five-spice powder
½ tsp sweetener
1 tsp sea salt
1 tsp ground black pepper
½ tsp chilli flakes
½ tsp white pepper

*Lining your meal prep
containers with baking
paper will stop the chips
going too soggy when
you reheat them.*

A firm favourite with our followers, these fries were originally inspired by the fact that I love chips and anything that goes with them. This dish is so tasty that Charlotte and I have been known to fight over it! So make sure you make plenty of portions!

1 Slice the potatoes into wedges, leaving the skin on as it tastes so great. Cook the wedges in a pan of salted boiling water for 5 minutes. Meanwhile, preheat the oven to 200°C and line a baking tray with baking paper.

2 Drain the chips and pat them dry with a tea towel or some kitchen roll. Tip them on to the lined baking tray and spray them liberally with low-cal spray.

3 Combine the ingredients for the spice mix together in a bowl and add a third of it to the chips, ensuring that they're all thoroughly coated. Cook the chips in the oven for 25–30 minutes until they're golden brown.

4 Whilst the chips are cooking, finely slice the red and green peppers. Heat the vegetable oil in a frying pan over a medium heat, then add the sliced peppers and the mince along with another third of the spice mixture. Cook for 3–5 minutes, adding the mince in batches so it browns evenly.

5 Once the wedges are cooked, sprinkle over the remaining spice mix and divide them between two baking paper-lined airtight containers. Add the mince mixture and top with the grated cheese. This will keep in the fridge for up to 3 days or in the freezer for up to 3 months.

6 If you're eating straight away, sprinkle the wedges with the cheese and put them back in the oven for 5 minutes so the cheese melts. Add the spring onions, peppers and a drizzle of sriracha sauce, if using.

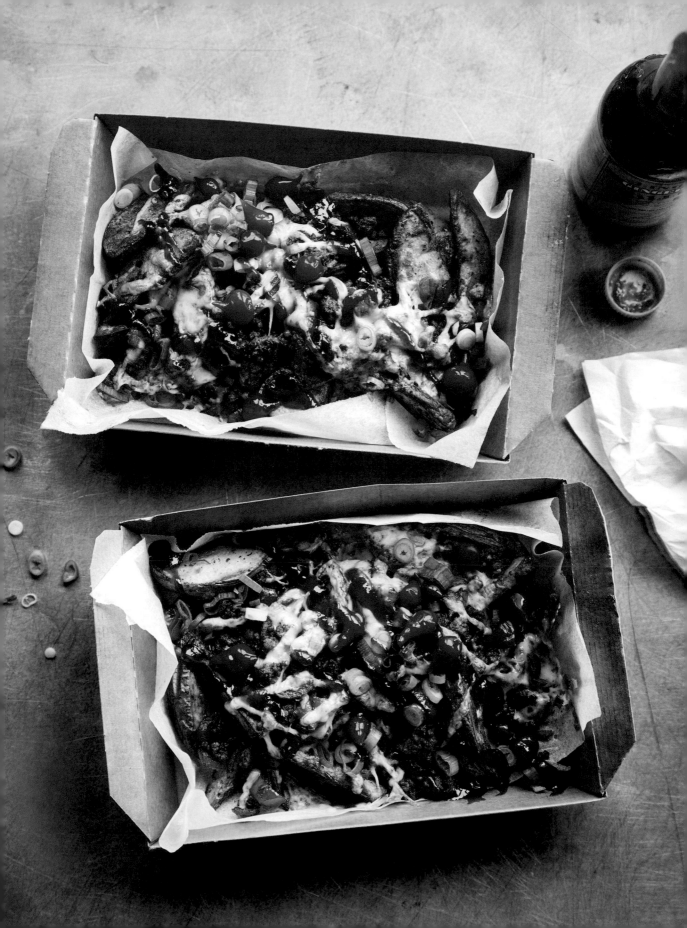

ONE-POT CHORIZO & CHICKPEA STEW

PER SERVING | **479** CALS | **22G** PROTEIN | **20G** FAT | **45G** CARBS

prep *cook* ❄

10 MINS   20 MINS   FREEZE

SERVES 2

1 tbsp olive oil
1 red onion, diced
2 cloves of garlic,
   peeled and crushed
50g chorizo sausage
300g cherry tomatoes
150g courgettes
1 x 400g tin of
   chickpeas, drained
1 tsp smoked paprika
1 tsp ground cumin
½ tsp ground coriander
1 tsp brown sugar
1 x 200g tin of sweetcorn,
   drained
½ tbsp tomato purée
1 vegetable stock cube
1 bay leaf
a small handful of fresh
   flat-leaf parsley,
   finely chopped
100g spinach
salt and pepper

To serve:
2 wholegrain pitta breads

This is another one of those dishes I put together using leftovers that has become a staple in our house. The smokiness from the chorizo and paprika mixed with the sweetness of the tomatoes and brown sugar combines in this stew nicely.

1 Heat the olive oil in a saucepan over a medium heat, add the onion and garlic and sauté for 3–5 minutes. Chop the chorizo sausage into small cubes, add to the pan and cook for a further 3–5 minutes.

2 Slice the cherry tomatoes in half and chop the courgettes into 5cm squares, then add to the pan along with the chickpeas. Stir in the smoked paprika, cumin, coriander and brown sugar.

3 Add the sweetcorn and tomato purée, crumble in the stock cube and add 200ml water, then season to taste. Add the bay leaf and simmer for 8–10 minutes (you can simmer this for longer whilst you're prepping other meals if you like) until the sauce has thickened.

4 Take the pan off the heat and remove the bay leaf. Stir in the chopped parsley and the spinach until wilted. Divide the stew between two airtight containers. It will keep for up to 3 days in the fridge or 3 months in the freezer. Delicious on its own or served with wholegrain pitta breads (don't forget to bear in mind the extra calories).

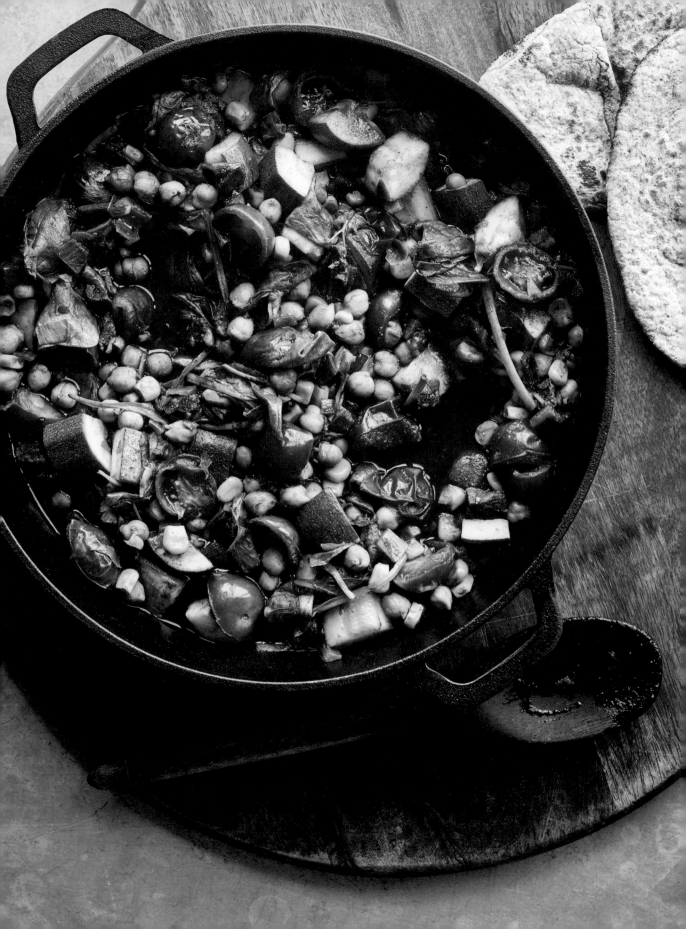

SPICY BEEF ENCHILADAS

PER SERVING | 492 CALS | 34G PROTEIN | 10G FAT | 58G CARBS

prep cook FREEZE
10 MINS 45 MINS

SERVES 2

1 tbsp sunflower oil
1/2 an onion, finely diced
150g 5% fat lean beef mince
1/2 tsp ground cumin
1/2 tsp hot chilli powder
1/2 tsp garlic salt
1 tsp dried mixed herbs
1 x 400g tin of kidney
    beans, drained
500g passata
a handful of fresh
    coriander, leaves picked
    and roughly chopped
4 mini tortillas
50g grated low-fat cheese
optional: fresh chillies,
    finely sliced
salt and pepper

*I like to add some of the
tinned juice from the kidney
beans to the mixture to
add more flavour. Try it!*

*There's something about homemade Mexican beef enchiladas
that I absolutely love. Deliciously spicy and cheesy, these
enchiladas are guaranteed to please the whole family.*

1 Heat the sunflower oil in a frying pan over a medium heat
and gently fry the onion for 8–10 minutes until soft. Add the
mince a bit at a time and brown for 2–3 minutes.

2 Add the cumin, hot chilli powder, garlic salt, mixed herbs,
kidney beans, 300g of the passata and give the mixture a good
stir, then season to taste. Leave it to simmer for 20 minutes,
stirring occasionally. Once the sauce has reduced, stir in the
chopped coriander leaves.

3 If you're meal prepping for later, divide the mixture between
the four mini tortillas and put two in each meal prep container.
Pour 100g of passata over each container and top with the
grated cheese. When you reheat them, the cheese will melt.
They will keep in the fridge for 3 days or in the freezer for
up to 3 months.

4 If you're eating straight away, preheat the oven to 200°C,
divide the mixture between the four mini tortillas and place
them in an ovenproof dish. Pour the passata over the tortillas
and sprinkle over the cheese. Bake them in the oven for 25–30
minutes until the cheese is golden brown. Sprinkle with some
more roughly chopped coriander if you have any spare. I like
to top these with loads of fresh chillies for that extra kick!

TURKEY & VEGETABLE JALFREZI WITH FRAGRANT RICE

PER SERVING | 475 CALS | 46G PROTEIN | 8G FAT | 51G CARBS

**15 MINS
+
MARINATING**   **30 MINS**   **FREEZE**

SERVES 2

300g lean turkey steaks
100g fat-free natural yoghurt
75g rice
4 cardamom pods
1 tbsp olive oil
2 green peppers, deseeded
1 onion, peeled
1 tsp chopped garlic
1 tsp chopped ginger
1 red chilli, deseeded
    and finely chopped
1 x 400g tin of chopped
    tomatoes (If you want a
    smoother texture, blend
    in a food processor)
a small bunch of fresh
    coriander, leaves and
    stalks finely chopped
salt and pepper

For the curry powder (or use a ready-made mix, to taste):
1 tsp ground turmeric
1 tsp ground coriander
a pinch of chilli powder
½ tsp ground cumin
1 tsp smoked paprika
½ tsp onion salt

*It's best to freeze or
refrigerate cooked rice
as soon as it's cooled. It'll
keep in the fridge for 1 day.
Do not reheat cooked rice
more than once.*

Tomatoes are your best friend when it comes to keeping calories low whilst still enjoying the foods you love. This curry is so easy to make and adding turkey to it is a nice touch.

1 Combine the ingredients for the curry powder together in a bowl. Chop the turkey steaks into chunks, then place in another bowl with half the curry powder and the yoghurt and stir to coat. Cover and put in the fridge for 1 hour.

2 Preheat the oven to 200°C. Place your marinated turkey chunks on a lined baking tray and cook for 10–12 minutes.

3 Cook the rice according to the packet instructions. Crush some cardamom pods and add to the cooking water for really fragrant rice.

4 Heat the olive oil in a saucepan over a medium heat. Slice the peppers and onion into thin strips and fry for 8–10 minutes, stirring occasionally, until they begin to soften. Add the garlic, ginger and chilli along with the rest of the curry powder and cook for 2–3 minutes more.

5 When the turkey is very nearly cooked, add it to the pan along with the tomatoes. Stir, cover and simmer for 5 minutes, stirring occasionally. If the sauce is too thick, add a splash of water. Season to taste, then add the chopped coriander and stir through the curry.

6 Divide the rice and curry between two airtight containers. It will keep for up to 1 day in the fridge or up to 3 months in the freezer.

BUTTER BEAN & VEGETABLE BIRYANI

PER SERVING | 455 CALS | 16G PROTEIN | 8G FAT | 72G CARBS

15 MINS   30 MINS   FREEZE

SERVES 2

1 tbsp olive oil
1 onion, finely diced
1 tsp chopped garlic
1 tsp chopped ginger
1 red pepper, finely sliced
100g green beans, halved
1 carrot, peeled and diced
1 stick of celery, diced
1/2 x 400g tin of
   chopped tomatoes
1 x 400g tin of butter
   beans, drained and rinsed
100g uncooked basmati
   rice, washed thoroughly
1 vegetable stock cube
salt and pepper

For the spice mix:
1/2 tsp ground cumin
1 tsp ground turmeric
1/2 tsp ground coriander
1 tsp garam masala
1/2 tsp cayenne pepper
1/4 tsp ground nutmeg
salt and pepper

To serve:
1 lime, cut into wedges

An exceptionally cheap but tasty meal prep which freezes perfectly, reheats a treat and contains a huge range of nutritious ingredients: beans, vegetables and turmeric, to name just a few. Traditionally, ghee is used to cook a lot of Indian food, but we're cutting this out to save on calories. It still tastes good though!

1 Combine the spices in a bowl. Heat the olive oil in a large saucepan over a medium heat. Sauté the onions for 2–3 minutes, then add the garlic, ginger and half the spice mix. Fry for 1 minute until the spices are fragrant.

2 Add the pepper, green beans, carrot and celery to the pan and cook for 4–5 minutes over a low heat, stirring regularly.

3 Add the tomatoes, butter beans, rice and the rest of the spice mix, crumble in the stock cube and add 200ml of water.

4 Simmer for 20 minutes with a lid on, stirring occasionally to stop the rice sticking to the bottom of the pan. Season to taste, add the lime wedges to squeeze over the top after you've reheated the meal, and divide between two airtight containers. This will keep in the fridge for up to 1 day or in the freezer for up to 3 months.

Top tip: It's best to freeze or refrigerate rice as soon as possible after cooking it, once it's cooled down. It'll keep in the fridge for up to 1 day. When reheating, make sure it is steaming hot all the way through. Do not reheat cooked rice more than once.

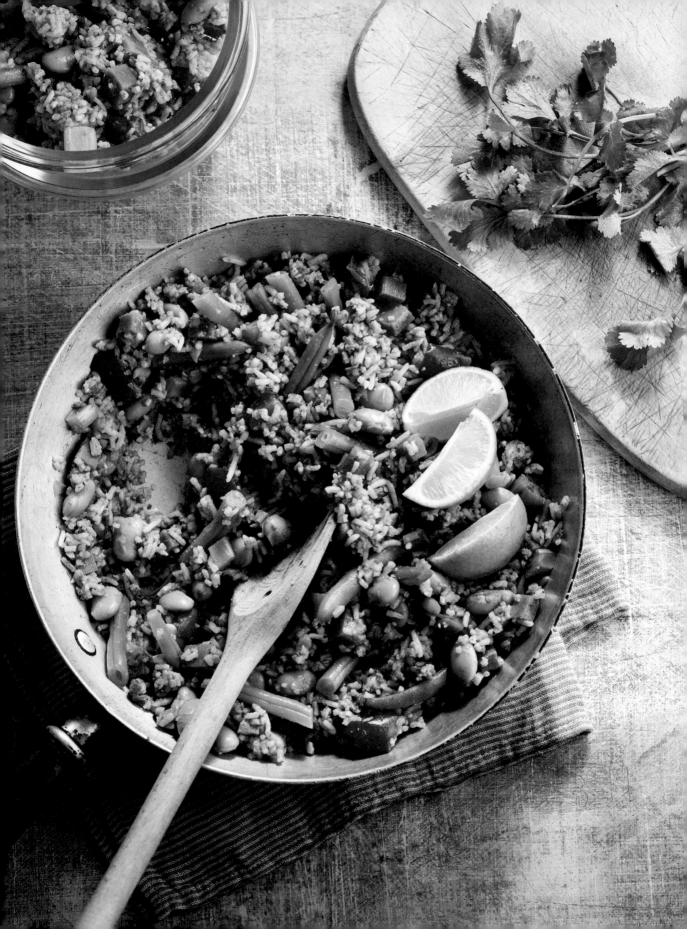

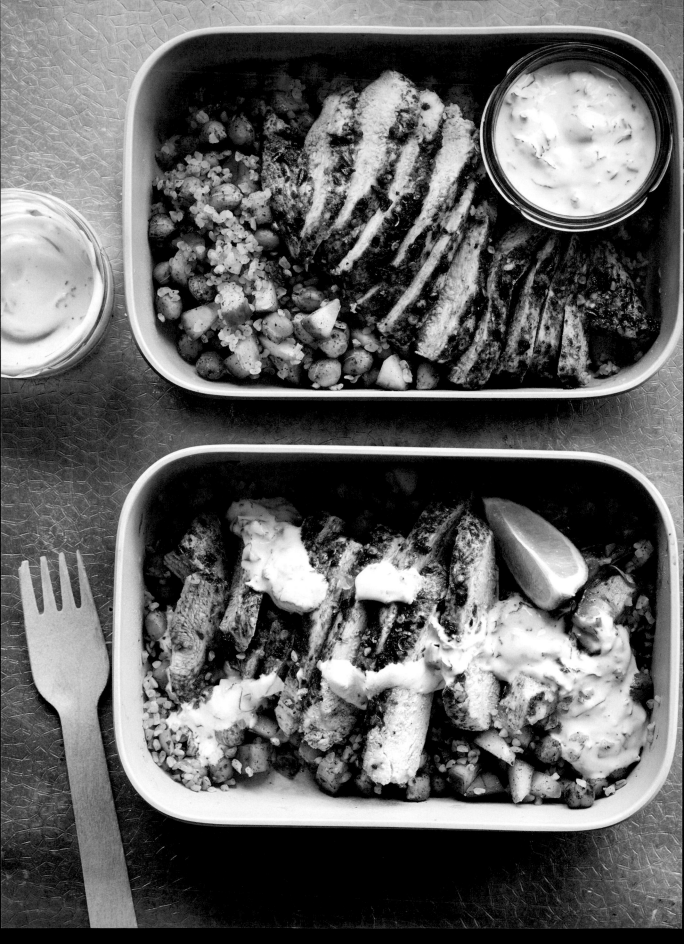

HARISSA CHICKEN & CHICKPEAS WITH BULGUR WHEAT

PER SERVING | **488** CALS | **43G** PROTEIN | **13G** FAT | **44G** CARBS

10 MIN   30 MINS

SERVES 2

2 chicken breasts (approx. 250g)
juice of 1 lemon
1 tbsp olive oil
2 tbsp harissa seasoning
    (see the recipe on page 33,
    or you can use ready-made)
1 x 400g tin of chickpeas,
    drained and washed
1 tsp smoked paprika
50g bulgur wheat
½ a cucumber, finely diced
salt and pepper

For the dressing:
100g fat-free yoghurt
1 clove of garlic, peeled
    and crushed
a small handful of fresh
    coriander, roughly chopped
salt and pepper

*Marinate your chicken
overnight in the fridge if
possible to enhance the
flavours even more! You can
cook the chicken as per the
method opposite and it will
keep in the freezer for up to
3 months. When you reheat
it, all you'll have to do is cook
the bulgur wheat, drain and
roast the chickpeas and
make the dressing.*

*This vibrant meal prep is bursting with flavours and has
a great kick to it. Chickpeas are so versatile and cheap,
that's why we use them in so many recipes.*

1 Put the chicken breasts between two sheets of baking
paper or clingfilm and bash with a rolling pin until they are
the same thickness all over (this ensures even cooking). Then
put the chicken breasts in an airtight container or a ziplock
food bag with half the lemon juice, the olive oil, harissa and
seasoning. Leave to marinate in the fridge for an hour
before cooking or overnight if possible.

2 Preheat the oven to 180°C. Spread the drained chickpeas
evenly on a baking tray and mix with the smoked paprika.
Roast in the preheated oven for 20 minutes until golden
brown. Meanwhile, cook the bulgur wheat according to
the packet instructions and drain.

3 Heat a frying pan until smoking hot and fry the chicken
for 1 minute on each side. Remove from the pan and wrap
in foil, then place on a baking tray and cook in the oven for
20–25 minutes. When you take the chicken out of the oven,
take it out of the foil straight away so it stops cooking.
Leave to stand for 5 minutes to ensure it's nice and juicy.

4 To make the yoghurt dressing, mix the remaining lemon
juice with the yoghurt, garlic and chopped coriander and
season to taste – divide between two small pots.

5 Divide the diced cucumber, bulgur wheat and roasted
chickpeas between two airtight containers and top each
one with a chicken breast. Add the dressing pots and
cover. They will keep in the fridge for 3 days.

SPAGHETTI & MEATBALLS

PER SERVING | 486 CALS | **25G** PROTEIN | **21G** FAT | **45G** CARBS

prep
15 MINS

cook
45 MINS

SERVES 2

50g beef mince
50g pork mince
30g breadcrumbs
20g Parmesan cheese,
    grated
1 clove of garlic, peeled
    and crushed
a small handful of fresh
    flat-leaf parsley,
    roughly chopped
1 egg
1 tbsp olive oil
120g spaghetti
salt and pepper

For the sauce:
300g cherry tomatoes
1 tbsp olive oil
1/2 tsp onion salt
1/2 tsp garlic salt
a small handful of fresh basil

*For a really good flavour,
add a spoonful of pesto
to the meatball mix – it
tastes great! You can cook
the meatballs and tomato
sauce as per the method
and it will keep in the
freezer for up to 3 months.
When you reheat it, all
you'll have to do is cook
the spaghetti.*

*A true Italian classic you won't want to miss! Once you've
made this tomato sauce, you'll never want to buy ready-
made sauce again.*

1 To make the sauce, preheat the oven to 200°C. Halve the
cherry tomatoes and spread them out on a baking tray. Drizzle
with the olive oil and sprinkle with the onion salt, garlic salt,
salt and pepper. Roast for 15–20 minutes until the tomatoes
start to colour and release their juices.

2 Allow the roasted tomatoes to cool, then tip into a food
processor, making sure you get all the juices from the tray.
Blend until smooth and then stir in the chopped basil (don't
blend it in – it will turn your sauce green!). Set to one side.

3 Mix the beef and pork mince, breadcrumbs, cheese,
garlic, most of the parsley and the egg together, season
and combine thoroughly.

4 Divide the mixture into eight meatballs. Heat a frying pan
over a medium heat, add the olive oil and brown the meatballs
on all sides for 15 minutes. Then pour in the tomato sauce,
cover and simmer for about 10 minutes, stirring occasionally.

5 Meanwhile, cook the pasta according to the packet
instructions, and don't forget to season it. Drain and mix into
the meatball sauce, ensuring it's fully coated. Then sprinkle
over the remaining chopped parsley before serving. This
will keep in the fridge for up to 3 days.

COURGETTI BOLOGNESE

PER SERVING | **494** CALS | **49G** PROTEIN | **23G** FAT | **19G** CARBS

prep 5 MINS **cook** 55 MINS

SERVES 2

650g cherry tomatoes
30ml olive oil
2/3 tsp onion salt
2/3 tsp garlic powder
10g basil leaves, roughly torn, plus extra for garnishing
300g lean turkey mince
1 onion, finely diced
2 medium courgettes
salt and pepper

If you don't have a spiralizer, you can always use a vegetable peeler and then slice the ribbons with a knife. You can cook the Bolognese as per the method and it will keep in the freezer for up to 3 months. When you reheat it, all you'll have to do is spiralize the courgettes.

This lean Bolognese is a low-carb option but you can always swap out the courgetti if you want to increase the carbs. Leave the courgette raw – when you heat it up, it won't be soggy!

1 Preheat the oven to 200°C. Halve the cherry tomatoes, then spread them evenly on a baking tray. Drizzle with half the olive oil and half the onion salt and garlic powder. Season well and roast in the oven for 35 minutes.

2 Tip the roasted tomatoes into a food processor and add the remaining onion salt and garlic powder along with the basil leaves. Blend to a smooth paste and set to one side.

3 Heat a frying pan over a medium heat and fry the turkey mince and onion with the remaining olive oil for about 10–12 minutes until cooked through. Season to taste. Add the tomato sauce to the pan and simmer for 10 minutes.

4 Spiralize the courgettes and divide between two airtight containers. It's best to leave the courgette raw if you're going to keep the meal in the fridge so that it won't be soggy when you reheat it. But if you want to eat the Bolognese straight away, heat half a tablespoon of olive oil in a hot frying pan and fry the courgetti for 30 seconds–1 minute.

5 Divide the tomato sauce equally between the two airtight containers and top with extra basil leaves. This will keep in the fridge for 3 days.

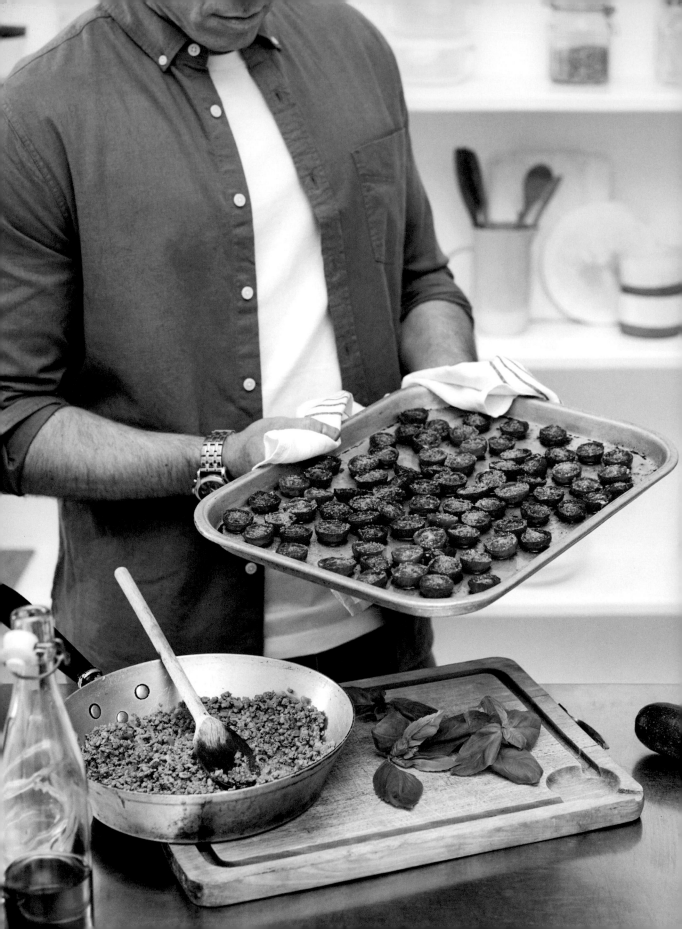

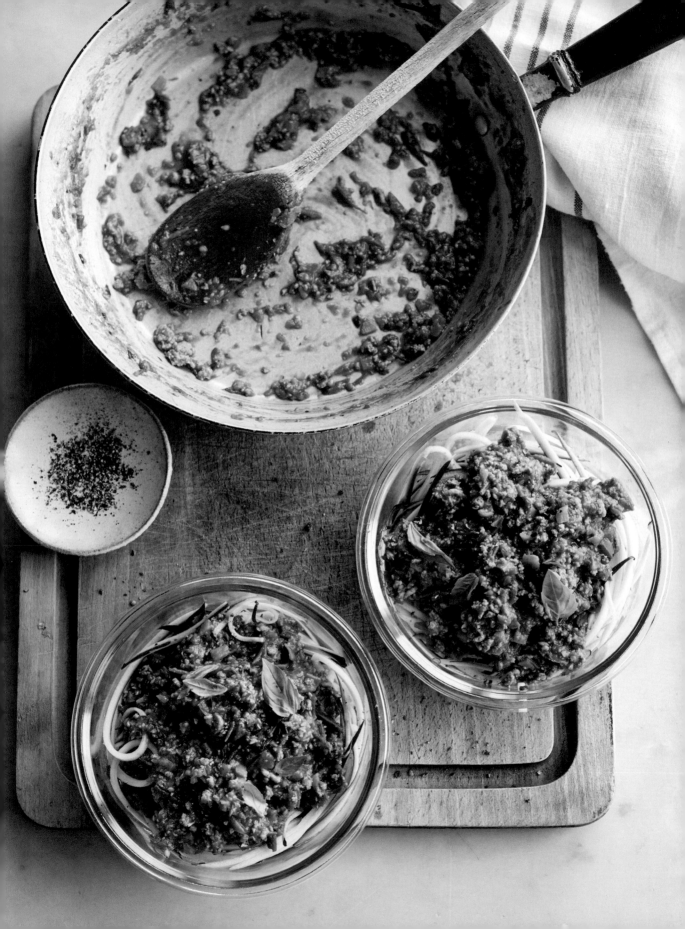

BEEF STIR-FRY WITH BLACK BEAN SAUCE

PER SERVING | 456 CALS | 36G PROTEIN | 13G FAT | 48G CARBS

prep 5 MINS   **cook** 15 MINS   **FREEZE**

SERVES 2

225g lean rump steak
1 tsp cornflour
1/2 tsp minced garlic
1/2 tsp minced ginger
1 tbsp olive oil
1/2 an onion, thinly sliced
1 red pepper, sliced
   into thin strips
1 red chilli, deseeded
   and finely sliced
75g sugar snap peas
75g baby corn, halved
1 tbsp soy sauce
120g packet of black
   bean sauce
250g packet of
   pre-cooked rice
1 spring onion, finely sliced

It's best to freeze or refrigerate rice as soon as possible after cooking it, once it's cooled down. It'll keep in the fridge for up to 1 day. When reheating, make sure it is steaming hot all the way through. Do not reheat cooked rice more than once.

Impress your family and friends with this extremely satisfying recipe that is ready in just 20 minutes. Feel free to add in any leftover vegetables that may be about to go off. Less waste, and you'll save money!

1 Remove any fat from the steak and slice it into thin strips. Lightly dust it with the cornflour in a bowl, tossing to coat, then add the garlic and ginger.

2 Heat the olive oil in a wok or frying pan over a medium heat. Add the onion and fry for 2–3 minutes. Then add the pepper and red chilli, reduce the heat and stir-fry for another 2–3 minutes. Remove from the pan and set to one side.

3 Put the steak in the same pan and fry it for 2–3 minutes, stirring continuously. Tip the onions, red peppers and chilli back into the pan and add the sugar snap peas and baby corn.

4 Stir in the soy sauce and the black bean sauce, ensuring that everything is fully coated, then fry over a low heat for a further 1–2 minutes.

5 Divide the cooked rice between two meal prep containers and top with the stir-fried meat and vegetables. It will keep in the fridge for 1 day or in the freezer for up to 3 months. If you're eating it right away, top with the thinly sliced spring onions.

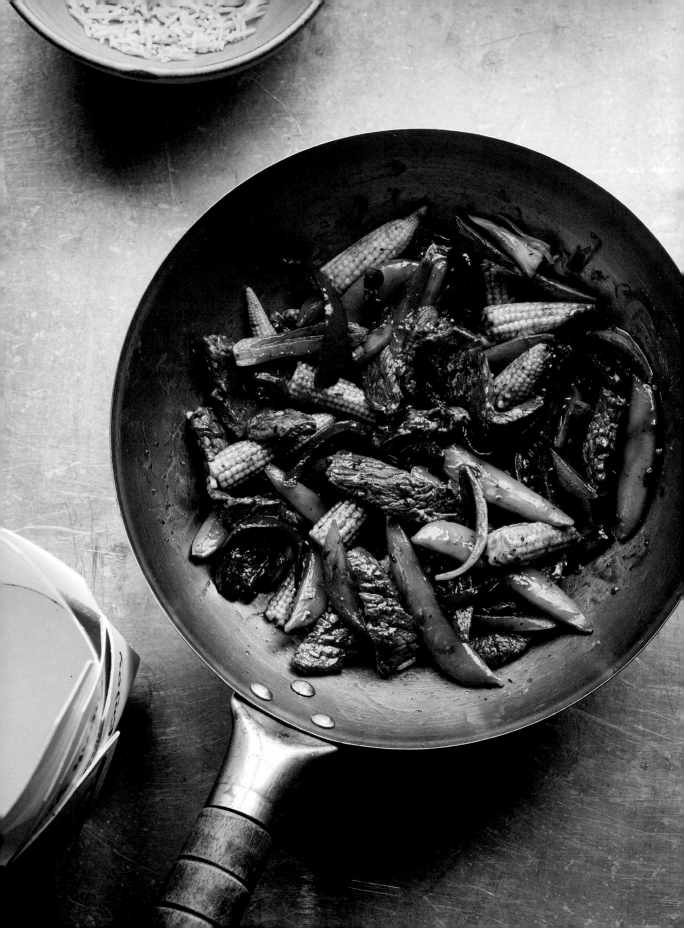

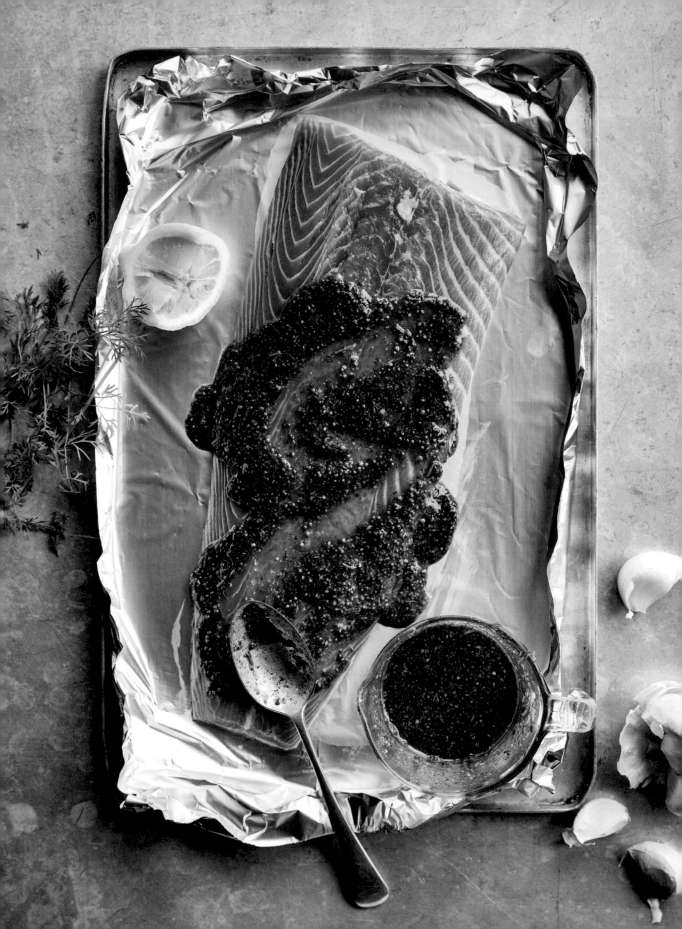

HONEY MUSTARD SALMON WITH POTATOES & GREEN BEANS

PER SERVING | **482** CALS | **38G** PROTEIN | **19G** FAT | **37G** CARBS

10 MINS   30 MINS   FREEZE
+RESTING

SERVES 4

½ a side of fresh salmon
  or 4 salmon fillets
  (about 600g in total)
2 cloves of garlic, peeled
  and crushed
a small handful of fresh dill,
  finely chopped
40g honey
50g wholegrain mustard
½ tsp paprika
juice of ½ a lemon
600g Charlotte potatoes
200g green beans
10g butter
a small handful of fresh
  parsley, finely chopped
salt and pepper

Another seafood favourite packed with some serious flavours. Using a side of salmon instead of individually packaged salmon fillets can save on cost as well.

1 Preheat the oven to 200°C. Put the salmon on a large sheet of foil. Mix the garlic, dill, honey, mustard, paprika, lemon juice and seasoning together in a bowl. Cover the salmon with the mixture, using a spoon to spread it over evenly. Wrap up the foil to form a parcel – not too tightly; leave room to add the green beans later on. Cook the salmon in the oven for 20 minutes.

2 Whilst the salmon is cooking, add the potatoes to a saucepan of boiling water for 15 minutes until tender.

3 Take the salmon out of the oven, add the green beans to the foil parcel and fold it back up. Put it back into the oven for 15 minutes.

4 Remove the salmon parcel from the oven and allow to rest for 5 minutes to firm up – then it's easier to portion out. Drain the potatoes and crush with the butter and chopped parsley. Divide between four airtight containers and top each one with a portion of salmon and some green beans. This will keep in the fridge for up to 3 days or in the freezer for up to 3 months.

CARIBBEAN PORK

PER SERVING | 472 CALS | 33G PROTEIN | 11G FAT | 56G CARBS

10 MINS   15 MINS   FREEZE

SERVES 2

200g pork fillet
    (or pork medallions)
1 tsp jerk seasoning (see the
    recipe on page 33, or you
    can use ready-made)
1 red onion
1 red pepper
1 yellow pepper
100g rice
1 tbsp olive oil
1 bird's-eye chilli, finely
    chopped
2 cloves of garlic, crushed
juice of 1 lemon
70g fresh pineapple, cut
    into bite-sized pieces
a handful of fresh flat-leaf
    parsley or coriander,
    roughly chopped
1 spring onion, sliced

*It's best to freeze or
refrigerate rice as soon
as possible after cooking it,
once it's cooled down. It'll
keep in the fridge for up
to 1 day. When reheating,
make sure it is steaming
hot all the way through.
Do not reheat cooked
rice more than once.*

*I absolutely love pork, it's full of protein and is naturally low
in fat. This recipe uses a cheap cut that stays juicy during
cooking. An easy mid-week dinner with a tropical twist!*

1 Thinly slice the pork fillet into bite-sized pieces, put in an
airtight container and cover with the jerk seasoning. Leave
to marinate in the fridge for an hour (you can leave it longer
if you wish).

2 Thinly slice the red onion, then deseed the peppers and
slice them into strips. Cook the rice according to the packet
instructions and drain.

3 Heat the olive oil in a frying pan over a medium heat.
Fry the pork for 2–3 minutes until browned, then remove
and set aside. Fry the onion and peppers in the same pan
for 8–10 minutes, stirring occasionally.

4 Stir in the chilli, garlic, lemon juice and pineapple and
cook for 1–2 minutes. Return the pork to the pan for the
last 60 seconds.

5 Divide the rice between two airtight containers and
top with the pork. If you're eating straight away, sprinkle
over the chopped parsley and sliced spring onion. This
will keep in the fridge for up to 1 day or in the freezer
for up to 3 months.

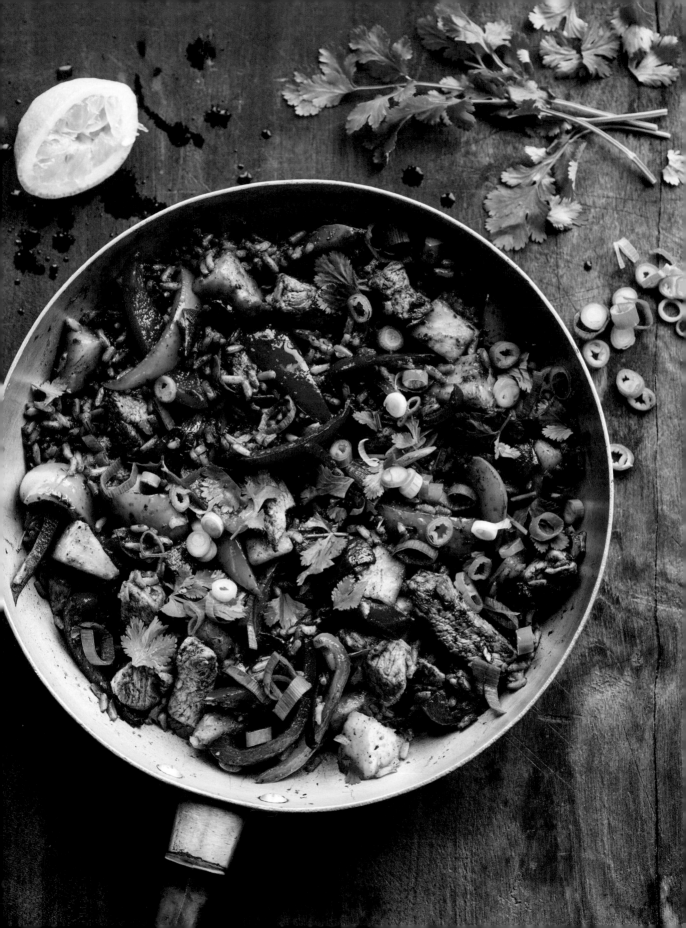

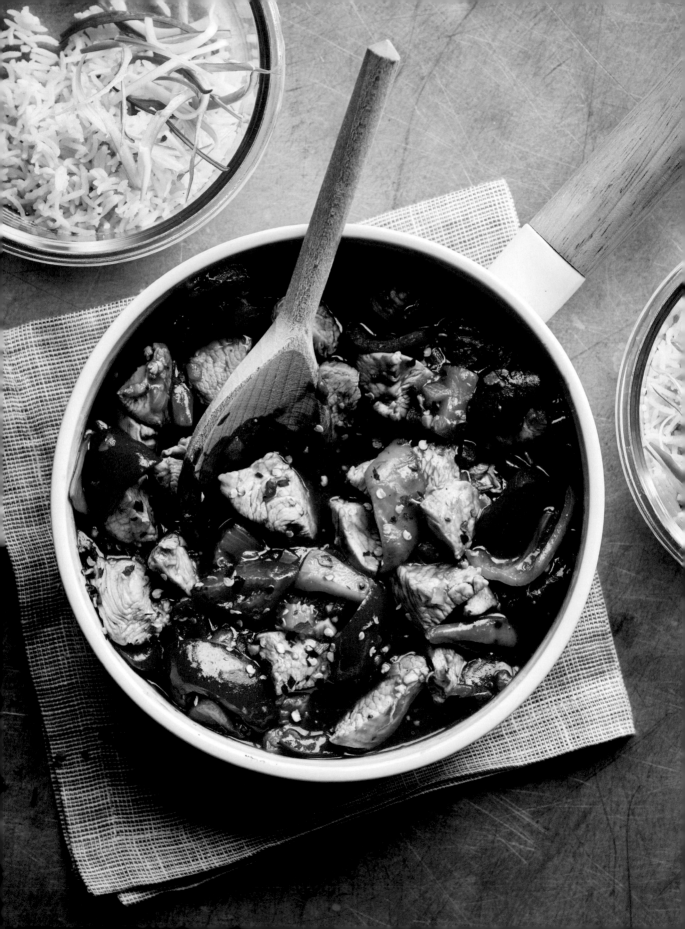

SWEET-AND-SOUR TURKEY

PER SERVING | **476** CALS | **46G** PROTEIN | **9G** FAT | **50G** CARBS

5 MINS   15 MINS   FREEZE

SERVES 2

2 turkey breasts
1 tbsp cornflour
1 tbsp sunflower oil
$^1/_2$ an onion, chopped
1 orange pepper, sliced
1 red pepper, sliced
$^1/_2$ tsp chopped garlic
1 tbsp tomato purée or
    tomato sauce
1 x 227g tin of pineapple
    chunks in juice
1 tbsp soy sauce
1 tbsp white wine vinegar
optional: juice of $^1/_2$
    an orange
125g packet of pre-cooked rice
salt and pepper
optional: 1 spring onion,
    sliced
optional: chilli flakes

*If you find the sauce isn't
thickening, whisk a teaspoon
of cornflour with 2–3
tablespoons of cold water
to create a paste. Mix it
into the sauce to thicken.*

*When reheating, make sure
it is steaming hot all the
way through. Do not reheat
cooked rice more than once.*

*A typical fast-food favourite done the healthy way. Why
should you miss out on a weekend treat? What's even better
is you can have this healthier version any day of the week.*

1 Slice the turkey into bite-sized pieces and toss them in
a bowl with the cornflour, salt and pepper, ensuring that
they're thoroughly coated.

2 Heat the sunflower oil in a frying pan over a medium
heat and fry the onion and peppers for 5–8 minutes, stirring
occasionally, until they start to soften. Add the turkey and
fry it for 2–3 minutes.

3 Add the garlic, tomato purée or sauce, pineapple chunks
and their juice, soy sauce and white wine vinegar to the pan
and mix everything thoroughly. Bring to the boil, then cover
and simmer for 5 minutes until the sauce thickens. Add the
juice of half an orange for extra flavour if you wish.

4 Divide the rice between two airtight containers and top
with the turkey. If using, sprinkle over the sliced spring onion
and chilli flakes. It will keep in the fridge for up to 1 day or
in the freezer for 3 months.

SAUSAGE & VEGETABLE TRAYBAKE

PER SERVING | 494 CALS | **15G** PROTEIN | **37G** FAT | **22G** CARBS

5 MINS   35 MINS

SERVES 2

½ a red onion
1 red pepper
2 tbsp olive oil
½ a courgette
½ an aubergine
100g cherry tomatoes
4 sausages
a few sprigs of fresh thyme
2 cloves of garlic, peeled
   and chopped
1 tbsp balsamic vinegar
salt and pepper

This is probably one of the best money-saving meal preps and it's extremely versatile. Limp-looking vegetables that would otherwise be thrown out are perfect for this recipe. Don't throw limp veggies away – prep them instead!

1 Preheat the oven to 200°C. Cut the red onion into four wedges and cut the pepper in half, remove the seeds and white flesh, then chop into 2.5cm squares. Put them both into a roasting tin and drizzle with 1 tablespoon of the olive oil. Roast for 10 minutes.

2 Whilst the red onion and pepper are cooking, chop the courgette and aubergine into large chunks. Halve the cherry tomatoes.

3 Add these to the roasting tin along with the sausages, thyme sprigs and garlic. Drizzle with the remaining olive oil and the balsamic vinegar, then season with salt and pepper. Mix everything so it's all thoroughly coated.

4 Roast for 25 minutes, stirring halfway through, until the vegetables are tender and the sausages are golden brown and fully cooked. Divide between two airtight containers. This will keep in the fridge for up to 3 days or in the freezer for up to 3 months.

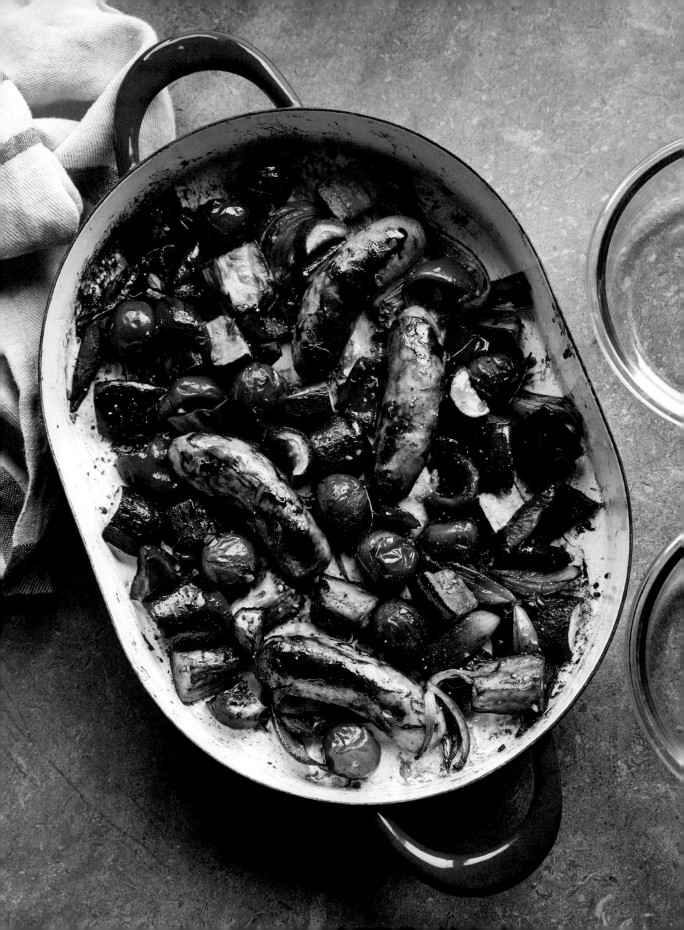

CHICKEN PARMESAN

PER SERVING | **497** CALS | **43G** PROTEIN | **23G** FAT | **27G** CARBS

prep 5 MINS **cook** 35 MINS **FREEZE**

SERVES 2

1 chicken breast
    (about 250g in total)
25g plain flour
1 egg
30g panko breadcrumbs
20g Parmesan cheese,
    grated
low-cal spray oil
50g grated mozzarella
50g cherry tomatoes
a small handful of fresh
    basil, roughly chopped
salt and pepper

For the sauce:
300g cherry tomatoes
1 tbsp olive oil
1/2 tsp onion salt
1/2 tsp garlic salt
a small handful of fresh
    basil, roughly chopped

This classic Italian dish should please even the fussiest of appetites. It's really great served on a bed of spinach, if you want to add more greenery to your plate.

1 To make the sauce, preheat the oven to 200°C. Halve the cherry tomatoes and spread them out on a baking tray. Drizzle with the olive oil and sprinkle with the onion salt, garlic salt, salt and pepper. Roast for 15–20 minutes until the tomatoes start to colour and release their juices.

2 Allow the roasted tomatoes to cool, then tip into a food processor, making sure you get all the juices from the tray. Blend until smooth and then stir in the chopped basil (don't blend it in – it will turn your sauce green!). Set to one side.

3 Slice the chicken in half horizontally. Put the flour in a bowl, season and stir. In another bowl, beat the egg. Mix the breadcrumbs and Parmesan in a third bowl and season.

4 Coat the chicken fillets in the flour, shake off any excess, then dip in the beaten egg and finally coat in the breadcrumbs, making sure the chicken is completely covered on both sides.

5 Line a roasting tin with baking paper and spray with low-cal spray. Roast the breadcrumbed fillets in the tin for 25 minutes, turning them over halfway, until golden brown.

6 If you're eating straight away, top the chicken with the mozzarella and return to the oven for 5 minutes so the cheese melts. If it's for meal prep, allow the chicken to cool and then add the cheese – it will melt when you reheat the meal.

7 Divide the tomato sauce between two airtight containers and add a piece of chicken to each one. Top with the cherry tomatoes and chopped basil. This will keep in the fridge for up to 3 days or in the freezer for up to 3 months.

SLOW-COOKER BEEF STEW

PER SERVING | **266** CALS | **33G** PROTEIN | **7G** FAT | **15G** CARBS

20 MINS **8 HOURS** **FREEZE**

SERVES 6

800g lean stewing steak
10g plain flour
1 onion
150g celery
200g Chantenay carrots
  (or normal carrots)
optional: 2 parsnips
1 tbsp olive oil
3 cloves of garlic
a sprig of fresh thyme
optional: 100g pickled
  onions (in a jar)
1 beef stock cube
1 bay leaf
3 tbsp Worcestershire
  sauce
1 x 400g tin of chopped
  tomatoes
salt and pepper

A slow cooker is an inexpensive asset to anyone looking to meal prep and it will become your secret weapon. You can leave this cooking overnight the day before you do all your meal prep so you already have six meals ready as soon as you wake up – a great head start!

1 Cut your beef into bite-sized cubes, place in a bowl, add the flour and mix to ensure all the beef is coated. Finely dice the onion and celery. Leave the Chantenay carrots whole (if you're using normal carrots, peel them and slice into rounds). Peel the parsnips, if using, cut in half widthways, then in half again.

2 Heat the olive oil in a saucepan over a medium heat and brown the beef for around 5 minutes, stirring to stop it sticking to the pan. Then set aside.

3 Finely chop the garlic and put it in the same pan the beef was cooked in along with the diced onion, celery and thyme. Fry over a low heat for about 5 minutes until the onion and celery are beginning to soften.

4 Put the vegetables into a slow cooker, along with the beef and the rest of the ingredients and 500ml of boiling water. Cook on a low setting for 8–10 hours (you can do this overnight), until the meat and vegetables are tender. If the stew looks too runny towards the end, take the lid off the slow cooker for an hour as this will allow the steam to escape and the stew to reduce.

5 Remove the bay leaf and divide the stew between six airtight containers. It will keep in the fridge for up to 3 days or in the freezer for up to 3 months.

COD & CHORIZO JAMBALAYA

PER SERVING | **367** CALS | **24G** PROTEIN | **7G** FAT | **49G** CARBS

prep **5 MINS** *cook* **40 MINS** **FREEZE**

SERVES 2

40g chorizo sausage
$1/2$ an onion, diced
1 green pepper, thinly sliced
1 clove of garlic, crushed
$1/2$ a stock cube
    (vegetable or chicken)
1 x 400g tin of chopped
    tomatoes
1 tsp Cajun seasoning (see
    the recipe on page 33, or
    you can use ready-made)
90g white rice
1 fillet of cod
a handful of fresh
    parsley, chopped
1 lime, cut into quarters
salt and pepper

It's best to freeze or refrigerate rice as soon as possible after cooking it, once it's cooled down. It'll keep in the fridge for up to 1 day. When reheating, make sure it is steaming hot all the way through. Do not reheat cooked rice more than once.

An irresistible Cajun-inspired dish using spicy Spanish sausage to add loads of flavour. Try adding more Cajun spice for an extra kick. How hot dare you make yours?

1 Chop the chorizo into bite-sized chunks. Heat a frying pan over a medium heat and add the chorizo to the pan. Fry the chunks for 2–3 minutes until they start to brown and release fat. Add the onion, pepper and garlic and fry for 8–10 minutes until they start to soften.

2 Pour 175ml of water into the pan along with the half stock cube, chopped tomatoes, Cajun seasoning and rice and stir everything together. Add the cod fillet to the pan, reduce the heat and cover with a lid. Leave it to simmer for 20–25 minutes until the water has been absorbed and the rice is cooked. Gently flake the cod into the mixture and stir to combine. Season to taste.

3 Sprinkle with chopped parsley and add a squeeze of lime juice. Divide between two airtight containers. This will keep in the fridge for up to 1 day or in the freezer for up to 3 months.

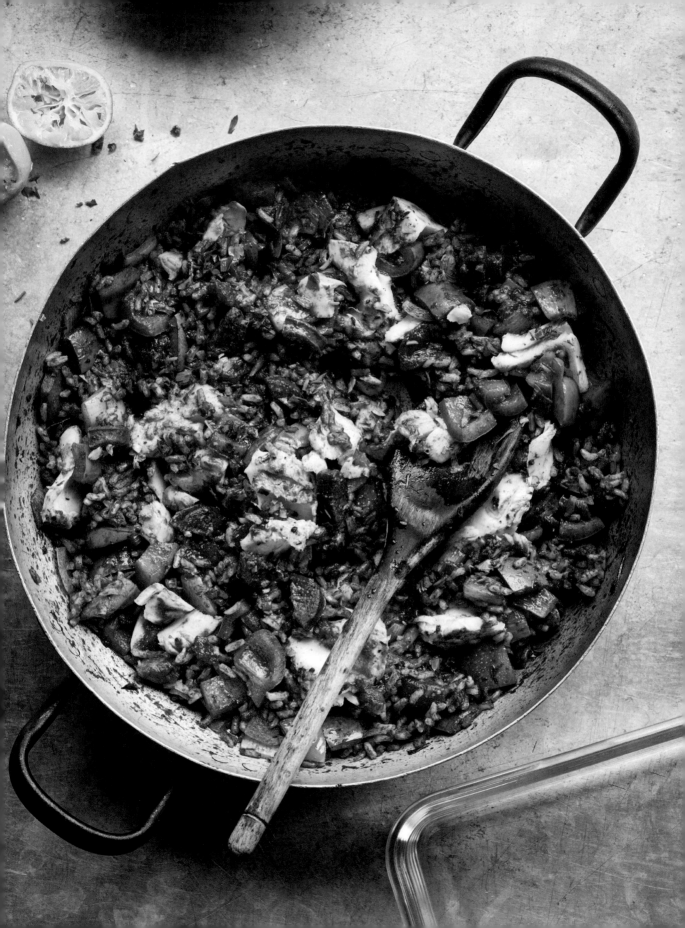

SLOW-COOKER BBQ PULLED CHICKEN

PER SERVING | **355** CALS | **25G** PROTEIN | **4G** FAT | **55G** CARBS

5 MINS   8 HOURS   FREEZE
30 MINS

SERVES 6

4 chicken breasts
250ml ketchup
2 tbsp mustard
2 tsp lemon juice
125ml honey
2 tbsp Worcestershire
  sauce
¼ tsp garlic granules
½ tsp chilli powder
¼ tsp cayenne pepper
1 tbsp brown sugar
salt and pepper
6 x 50g bread rolls

Meal prep and slow cookers go hand in hand. Switch it on the night before meal prep day if you want to save even more time in the kitchen. You'll be surprised how much time you can save just by organizing a few things the night before.

1 Place the chicken breasts in the bottom of a slow cooker along with 100ml of water. Mix the wet ingredients and the spices together along with the sugar and seasoning. Pour the sauce over the chicken.

2 Set the slow cooker to low and cook for 6–8 hours. When the chicken is cooked, shred it with a fork, mix it in with the sauce and season to taste. Leave to cook for a further 30 minutes.

3 If it's for meal prep, divide the chicken between six airtight containers. It will keep in the fridge for up to 3 days or in the freezer for up to 3 months. If you're eating straight away, serve the chicken spooned into the bread rolls.

CRISPY CHEESE & BACON POTATOES

PER SERVING | 500 CALS | 21G PROTEIN | 24G FAT | 48G CARBS

5 MINS 55 MINS

SERVES 2

500g potatoes,
   peeled and diced
low-cal spray oil
20g light margarine
1 tsp onion powder
1 tsp dried parsley
40ml ranch dressing
   or sour cream
75g low-fat Cheddar
   cheese
2 rashers of cooked
   streaky bacon, cut
   into bite-sized pieces
2 spring onions,
   finely sliced
optional: 2 handfuls of
   mixed salad leaves
salt and pepper

*This is a super-easy meal prep with loads of flavour that
reheats to perfection in the microwave. You'll be the envy
of everyone at work – they'll be wondering why they've gone
to a local shop for a lunchtime meal deal when in 3 minutes
you have this delicious meal for a fraction of the price.
I know which one I'd rather have.*

1 Preheat the oven to 190°C. Put the diced potatoes on a
baking tray, spray with low-cal oil and mix. Melt the margarine
and drizzle it over the potatoes. Then add the onion powder
and parsley and mix everything so it's well combined. Season
to taste.

2 Cover the baking tray with foil and roast the potatoes in
the oven for 20–25 minutes. Remove the foil and return the
potatoes to the oven for a further 25 minutes until they're
cooked and golden brown.

3 If you're going to eat straight away, add the ranch dressing
or sour cream, Cheddar cheese and bacon to the baking tray
and mix everything together. Put it back in the oven for a
further 10 minutes until everything has melted and it's golden
brown. Sprinkle over the chopped spring onions and enjoy!
Serve with mixed salad leaves if you like.

4 If it's for meal prep, divide the potatoes evenly between
two airtight containers and allow to cool. Then add the ranch
dressing or sour cream, Cheddar cheese and bacon. It will
keep in the fridge for up to 3 days. When you reheat it in the
microwave, the cheese will melt and it will taste delicious!
Sprinkle the sliced spring onions over the top and enjoy.

MAC & CHEESE

PER SERVING | **497** CALS | **22G** PROTEIN | **18G** FAT | **61G** CARBS

prep 15 MINS   **cook** 15 MINS   FREEZE

SERVES 2

75ml skimmed milk
20g light margarine
½ tsp yellow mustard
75ml low-fat sour cream
50g low-fat Cheddar
   cheese, shredded
10g grated Parmesan
   cheese
150g macaroni
1–2 tbsp fresh breadcrumbs
a small bunch of fresh
   flat-leaf parsley, chopped
salt and pepper
optional: 2 handfuls of
   mixed salad leaves

*For extra nutrients, add
a handful of raw spinach
to your meal prep
containers. When you
come to heat up the meal,
the spinach wilts and you
just mix it in. Delicious!*

*Can you ever have too much cheese? Of course you can't.
My take on this normally high-calorie favourite uses low-fat
alternatives to keep the calories down, but it still has all the
flavour. Enjoy!*

1 Preheat the oven to 200°C. In a large saucepan, combine
the milk, margarine, mustard, sour cream and the cheeses
along with a pinch of salt and pepper and cook over a low heat,
stirring, until everything is combined into a smooth sauce.

2 Cook the macaroni in salted water as per the packet
instructions and drain.

3 Mix the drained pasta into the cheese sauce. If you're
eating straight away, pour it into an ovenproof dish, sprinkle
over the breadcrumbs and cook it in the oven for 10–15 minutes
until the top is golden brown. Sprinkle over the chopped
parsley and serve with the mixed salad leaves, if using. If it's
for meal prep, divide the macaroni cheese evenly between
two airtight containers. It will keep in the fridge for up to
3 days or in the freezer for up to 3 months.

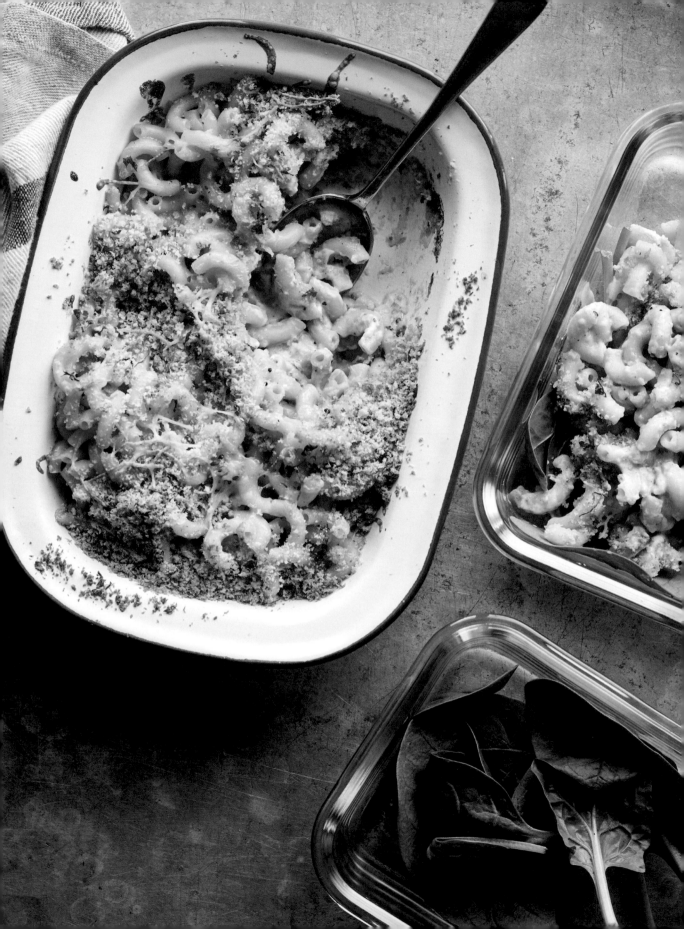

SAUSAGE & ROOT MASH WITH ONION GRAVY

PER SERVING | **494** CALS | **20G** PROTEIN | **17G** FAT | **61G** CARBS

5 MINS   30 MINS   FREEZE

SERVES 2

200g chicken sausages
15g butter
1 medium-sized onion,
    sliced
1 tsp brown or white sugar
1 tbsp plain flour
1 beef stock cube
150g sweet potatoes
150g potatoes
100g carrots
100g swede
30ml semi-skimmed milk
salt and pepper

Everyone loves 'bangers and mash'. You can also try adding some broccoli or cauliflower to the mash as it's a great way to include more vegetables in your diet. It doesn't all have to be about potatoes!

1 Preheat the oven to 200°C. Line a baking tray with foil and roast the sausages as per the packet instructions, turning occasionally, until they're golden brown.

2 Melt half the butter in a frying pan over a medium heat, add the sliced onion and sugar and fry for 10 minutes, stirring occasionally.

3 Add the flour to the caramelized onion, stir and cook for 30 seconds–1 minute. Sprinkle in the stock cube and pour in 400ml of water. Bring to the boil, then reduce the heat and leave to simmer for 10–15 minutes until it has thickened.

4 Peel and chop the potatoes and root vegetables into medium-sized cubes. Add to a pan of salted boiling water for 20–25 minutes until tender, then drain. Add the rest of the butter and the milk, mash until smooth and season to taste.

5 Divide the sausages and root mash between two airtight containers. Divide the gravy between two little sauce pots and slot into the containers. This will keep in the fridge for up to 3 days or in the freezer for up to 3 months.

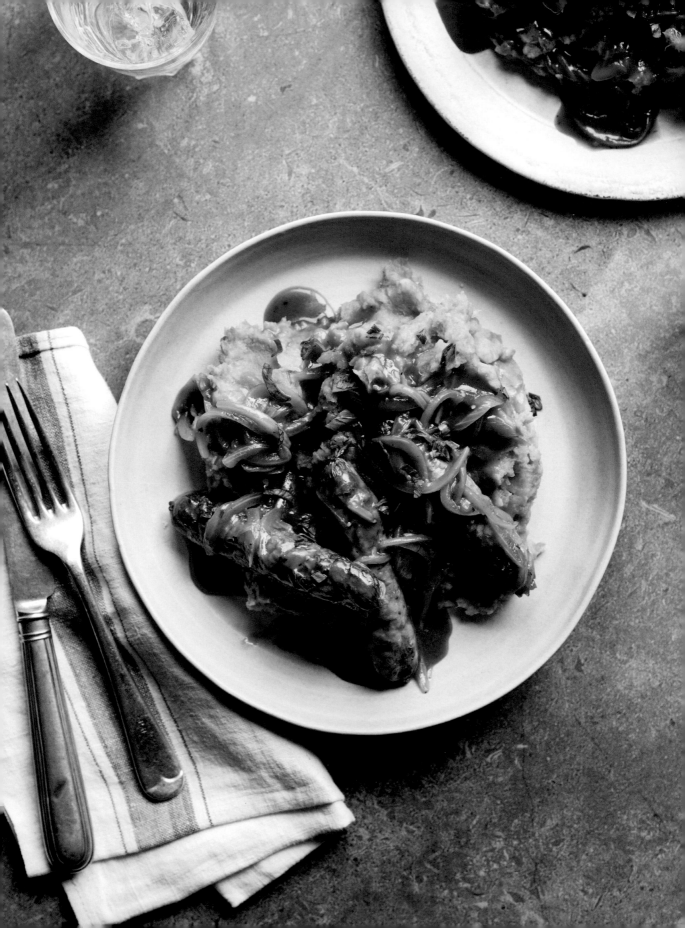

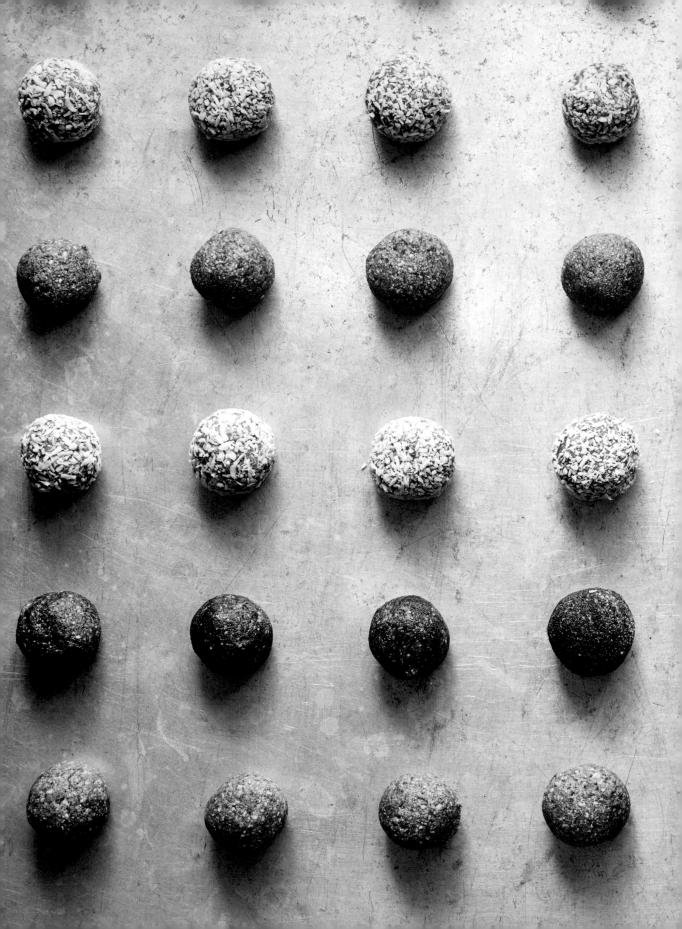

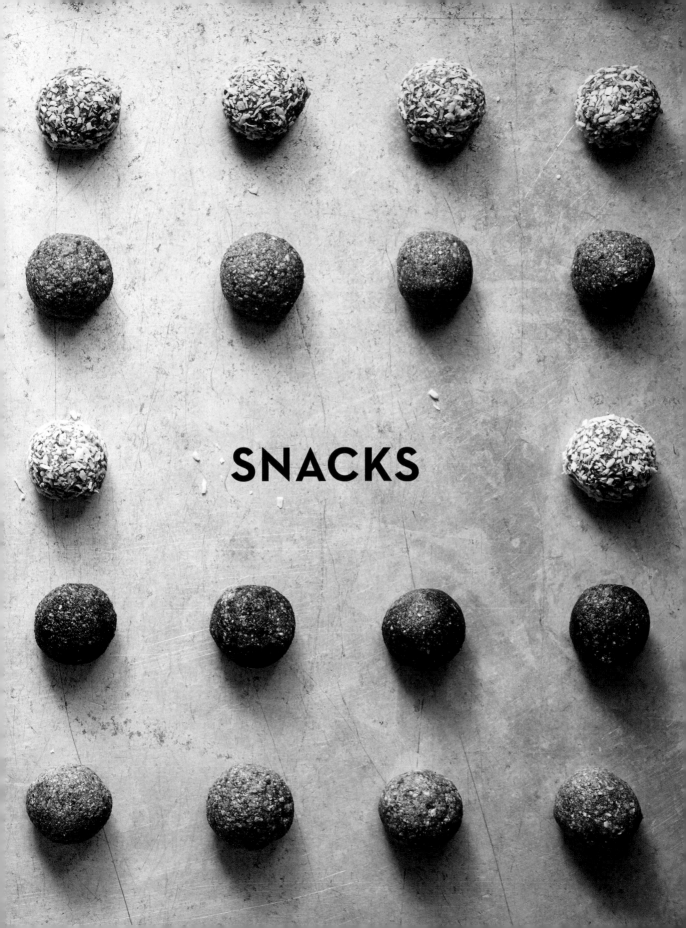

SNACKS

FRANK'S MALT BREAD

PER SERVING | **246 CALS** | **4G PROTEIN** | **1G FAT** | **54G CARBS**

PREP 10 MINS   **COOK** 55 MINS   **FREEZE**

SERVES 10

1 egg
approx. 140ml semi-
    skimmed milk
220g self-raising flour,
    plus ¹/₂ tbsp for dusting
¹/₂ tsp allspice
60g black treacle
90g golden syrup
60g malt extract
optional: 100g caster sugar
170g sultanas or raisins

tip

*If you want to reduce
the calories, you can cut
the sugar from this recipe
as it tastes just as good
without it!*

*Frank's malt bread is what he's best known for and he's very
proud of this recipe. It's always better the day after it's been
made and it's best enjoyed with butter and a cup of tea.
My absolute favourite afternoon snack!*

1 Preheat the oven to 180°C and line a loaf tin with baking paper.

2 In a jug, beat the egg and then pour in the milk.

3 Sift the self-raising flour into a bowl with the allspice. Then
add the black treacle, golden syrup, malt extract and sugar
(if using) along with the egg and milk mixture. Mix thoroughly,
ensuring that everything is well combined.

4 Dust the raisins with half a tablespoon of flour (this ensures
the fruit doesn't all sink to the bottom) and gently fold into
the mixture.

5 Pour the mixture into the loaf tin and bake on the bottom
shelf of the oven for 45 minutes. Then turn the oven down to
150°C and bake for an additional 20–25 minutes. To make sure
it's cooked, insert a skewer: if it comes out clean then the malt
bread's fully cooked. Leave to cool before eating. It will keep in
an airtight tin for 5–7 days or in the freezer for up to 3 months.

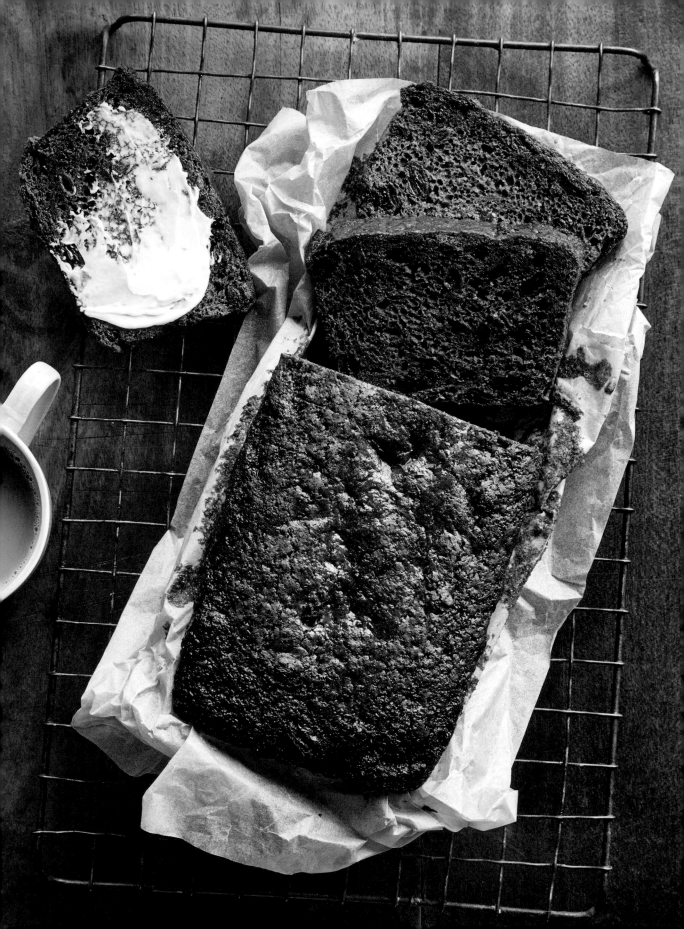

STORE-CUPBOARD BARS

PER SERVING | **180** CALS | **2G** PROTEIN | **10G** FAT | **20G** CARBS

5 MINS   20 MINS   FREEZE

MAKES 10 BARS

2 tbsp golden syrup/honey
50g brown sugar
100g butter
1/4 tsp salt
175g porridge oats

The reason I call these store-cupboard bars is because everyone tends to have these staple ingredients in their cupboard. They take very little time to make, cost pennies and are a great way to get your kids into the kitchen. They make a fantastic mid-afternoon snack or pre-workout treat.

1 Line a baking tray with baking paper and preheat the oven to 180°C.

2 In a large saucepan, over a low heat, melt the golden syrup or honey, sugar, butter and salt, stirring to combine until smooth. Add the oats and mix again so the oats are fully coated.

3 Tip the mixture into the lined baking tray and press it down with the back of a spoon so it's compact. Bake in the middle of the oven for 10–15 minutes until golden brown. Leave to cool and harden up before cutting into 10 bars. They will keep in an airtight container for up to 3 days or in the freezer for up to 3 months.

OATMEAL RAISIN COOKIES

PER SERVING | **167** CALS | **3G** PROTEIN | **6G** FAT | **24G** CARBS

15 MINS

15 MINS

FREEZE

MAKES 14 COOKIES

85g unsalted butter
100g brown sugar
1 tsp vanilla essence
1 egg
100g self-raising flour
150g oats
100g raisins

These are an excellent alternative to shop-bought cookies, and kids will love making them (as well as adults!). I use oats a lot as they're so good for you, packed with important vitamins, minerals and antioxidants.

1 Preheat the oven to 180°C. Mix together the butter, sugar and vanilla essence until pale and creamy. Then beat in the egg. Sift the flour into the mixture and add the oats and raisins.

2 Line two baking sheets with baking paper and place golfball-sized balls of the mixture on the trays, leaving 5cm between the cookies so they can spread when cooking. Flatten the balls down.

3 Bake the cookies for 15 minutes until golden brown, then leave to cool completely on a wire rack. They will keep in a sealed container for 5–7 days or in the freezer for up to 3 months.

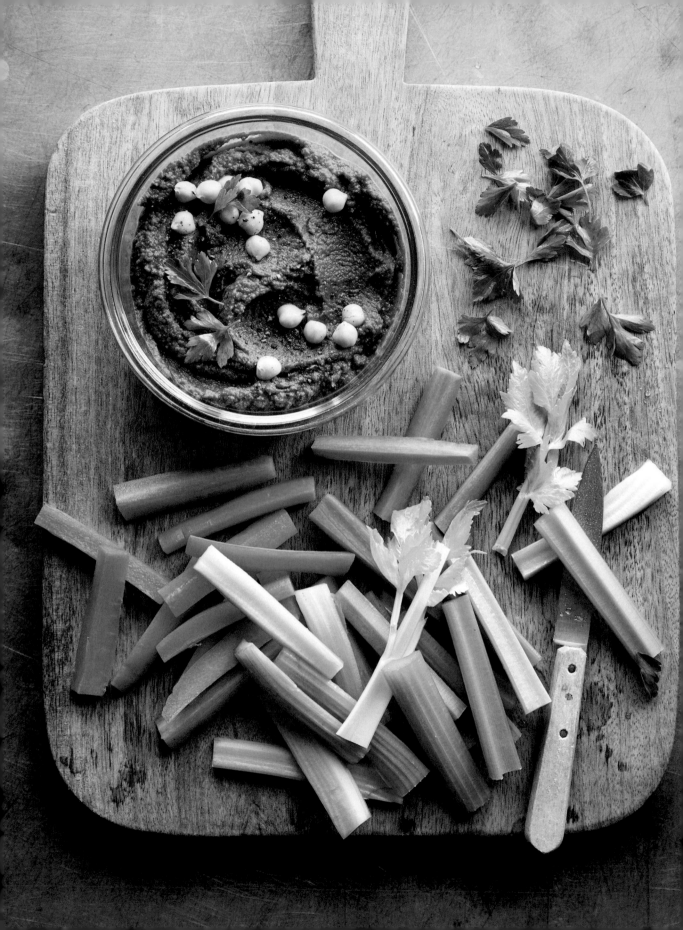

BEETROOT HUMMUS WITH CARROT & CELERY

PER SERVING | **155** CALS | **6G** PROTEIN | **5G** FAT | **18G** CARBS

15 MINS **45 MINS** **FREEZE**

SERVES 4

1 large beetroot (250g)
   or 1 packet of cooked
   beetroot (250g)
1 x 400g tin of chickpeas,
   drained
1 clove of garlic, peeled
juice of 1 lemon
1/2 tsp ground cumin
1/2 tsp sunflower seeds
1 tbsp olive oil
salt and pepper
optional: a small handful
   of fresh flat-leaf parsley,
   roughly chopped
2 carrots, peeled
3 sticks of celery

*I like to hold back
a few chickpeas so
I can stir them into the
hummus afterwards,
for added texture.*

*A super-simple recipe made with fresh tasty ingredients
and bursting with flavour. The colours alone will leave you
feeling refreshed!*

1 If you are roasting the beetroot, preheat the oven to 200°C.
Place the beetroot in a tray and drizzle with some olive oil,
then season. Roast for 40–45 minutes until tender. Leave to
cool, then peel off the skin, cut off the stalks and slice into
large chunks.

2 Put the beetroot, chickpeas, garlic, lemon juice, cumin,
sunflower seeds, olive oil and seasoning into a food processor
along with 1 tbsp of water. Blend until smooth.

3 Stir in the whole chickpeas, if you reserved some, as well
as the chopped flat-leaf parsley, if using. Chop your carrot
and celery into sticks and tuck in. The hummus will keep in the
fridge for up to 3 days or you can freeze it for up to 3 months.

SWEET POTATO BROWNIES

PER SERVING | **224** CALS | **6G** PROTEIN | **12G** FAT | **21G** CARBS

10 MINS   40 MINS   FREEZE

MAKES 9 BROWNIES

150g sweet potatoes
1 large egg
125g nut butter
  (I use almond)
120g honey
30g unsweetened
  cocoa powder
1/2 tsp baking powder
2 tsp vanilla extract
100g dark chocolate

*These are a super-quick, easy and cheap weekday treat.
I love to have one as an afternoon snack with a cup of tea
or to heat one up with some ice cream for a weekend treat.*

1 Peel and cut the sweet potatoes into large chunks. Bring
a pan of water to the boil and cook the sweet potatoes for
15–20 minutes until tender.

2 Preheat the oven to 180°C. Put the cooked sweet potatoes
in a food processor with the egg, nut butter, honey, cocoa
powder, baking powder and vanilla extract. Blend until smooth.

3 Line a baking tin (20cm x 20cm). Pour in the mixture, smooth
it out with a spatula and bake in the oven for 25–30 minutes
until set. To test that it's cooked through, poke in a skewer:
if it comes out clean, then it's ready.

4 Allow the brownies to cool in the tin for 15 minutes, then
remove and leave to cool completely. Melt the dark chocolate
(you can do this in short bursts in the microwave or in
a heatproof bowl over a saucepan of boiling water), then
spread it over the top of the cooled brownies and leave
to set. Cut the brownies into nine squares. They will keep
in an airtight container for up to 5 days or in the freezer
for up to 3 months.

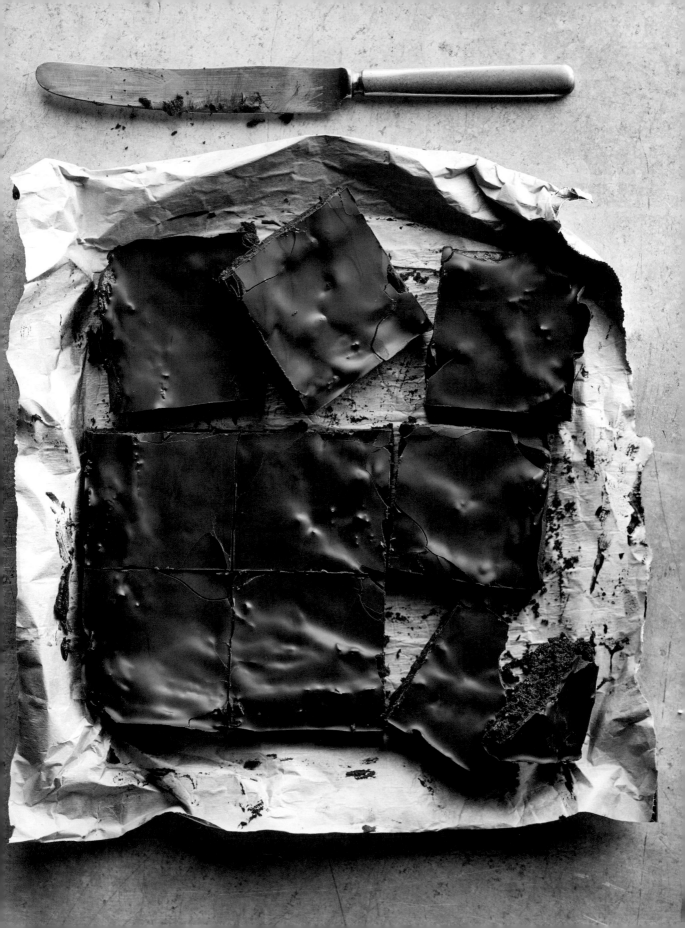

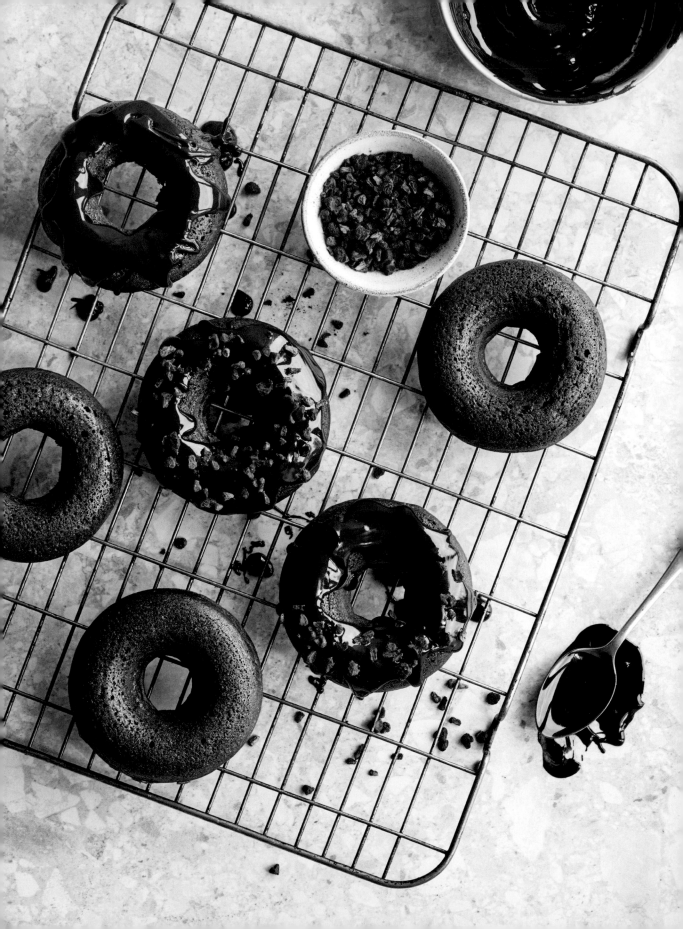

DOUBLE-CHOCOLATE PROTEIN DOUGHNUTS

PER SERVING | **156** CALS | **12G** PROTEIN | **5G** FAT | **15G** CARBS

15 MINS   15 MINS   FREEZE

MAKES 10 DOUGHNUTS

low-cal spray oil
130g wholegrain flour
300g 0% fat Greek yoghurt
2 large eggs
25g raw cacao powder
60g protein powder
1 tsp sweetener
1^{1}/2 tsp baking powder
84g dark chocolate
   (at least 70% cacao)
sprinkles to decorate

I love to have one of these doughnuts for a snack – at 156 calories a pop they're almost entirely guilt-free! Aren't they the best-looking low-calorie doughnuts you've ever seen? You will need to buy a doughnut tray but I can promise that you won't regret it.

1 Preheat the oven to 180°C and lightly grease your doughnut tray with the low-cal oil.

2 Mix all the ingredients (except the chocolate and sprinkles) thoroughly in a bowl, then divide the mixture equally between ten moulds.

3 Place on a middle shelf in the oven and cook for 10 minutes, then turn each doughnut over and cook for a further 5 minutes.

4 Whilst the doughnuts are baking, melt the chocolate (you can do this in short bursts in the microwave or in a heatproof bowl over a saucepan of boiling water).

5 Remove the doughnuts from the oven and the tray and leave them to cool on a rack. Cover the top of each doughnut with the melted chocolate and the sprinkles. The doughnuts will keep in a sealed container for 5–7 days or in the freezer for up to 3 months.

VEGETABLE CRISPS

PER SERVING | **81** CALS | **0G** PROTEIN | **6G** FAT | **6G** CARBS

5 MINS   15 MINS

SERVES 2

150g vegetable peelings
    (carrot, parsnip, beetroot
    and sweet potato)
1 tbsp olive oil
optional: $\frac{1}{2}$ tsp smoked
    paprika
optional: $\frac{1}{2}$ tsp curry
    powder

This is a fantastic way of using up vegetable peelings, to avoid food waste and save money!

1 Preheat the oven to 200°C and line a baking tray. Place the vegetable peelings in a bowl with the olive oil and season to taste. You can toss them in spices too, if you like.

2 Spread the vegetable peelings out on the lined baking tray, ensuring that they don't overlap. Bake for 15 minutes, turning halfway through, or until crisp. They will keep in an airtight container for up to a week.

SMOKY PAPRIKA POPCORN

PER SERVING | **165** CALS | **2G** PROTEIN | **12G** FAT | **12G** CARBS

15 MINS 3 MINS

SERVES 2

2 tbsp olive oil
40g popcorn kernels
1 tsp smoked paprika
a pinch of sea salt

Who doesn't love popcorn? It doesn't have to be a guilty pleasure though, thanks to my super-quick and easy recipe – perfect for film nights!

1 Heat 1 tablespoon of the olive oil in a large saucepan (with a lid) over a medium heat. Add the popcorn kernels, cover the pan and turn up the heat to high. Cook for 2–3 minutes, shaking occasionally, until all the popcorn has popped.

2 Put the popcorn into a sealable container and add the smoked paprika, the remaining olive oil and the salt. Seal and shake until the popcorn is evenly coated. It will keep for up to a week in an airtight container.

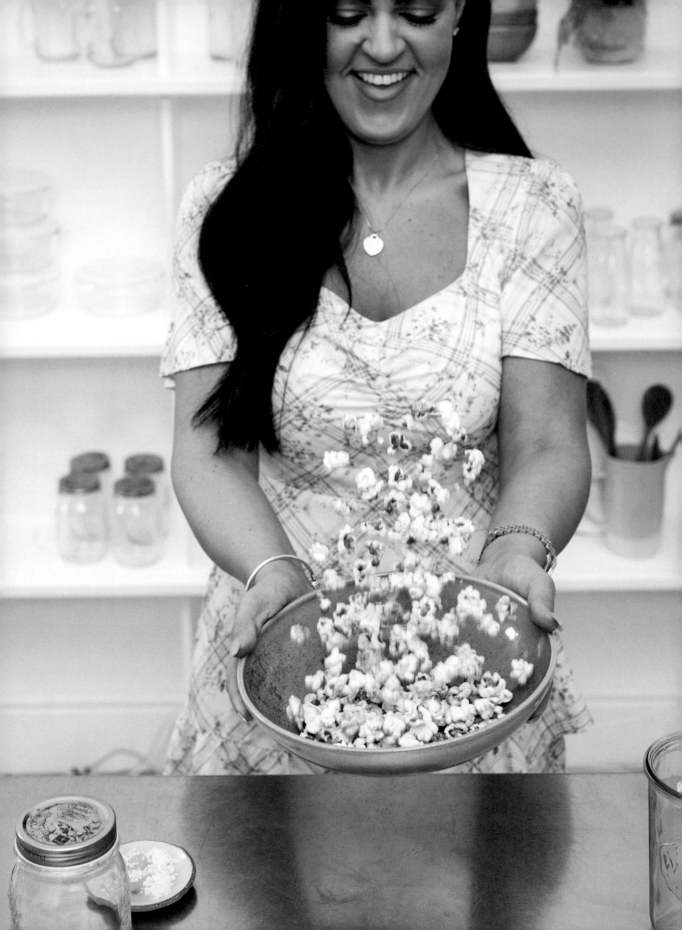

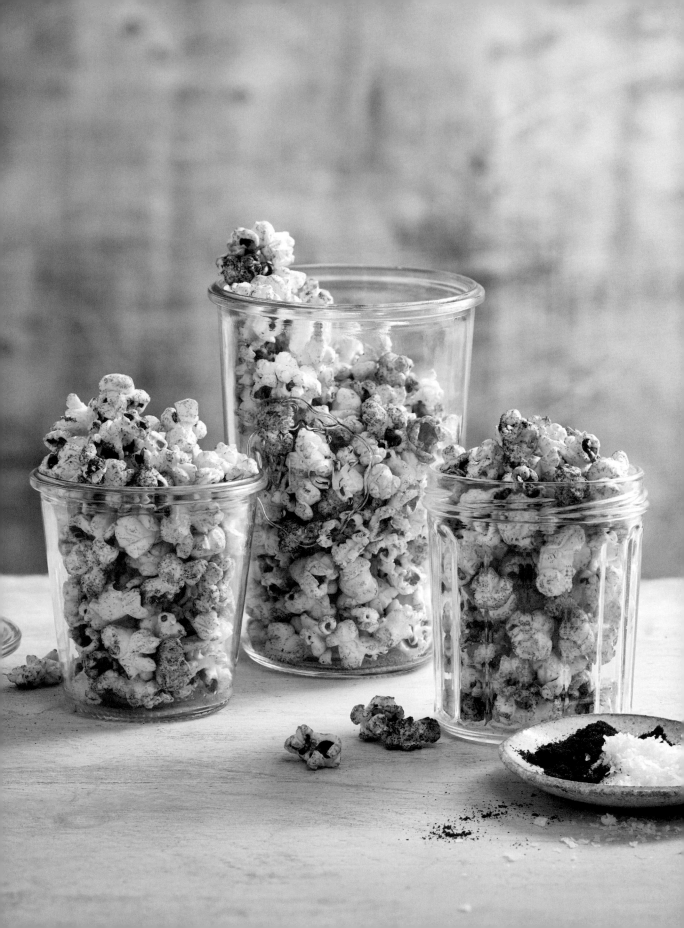

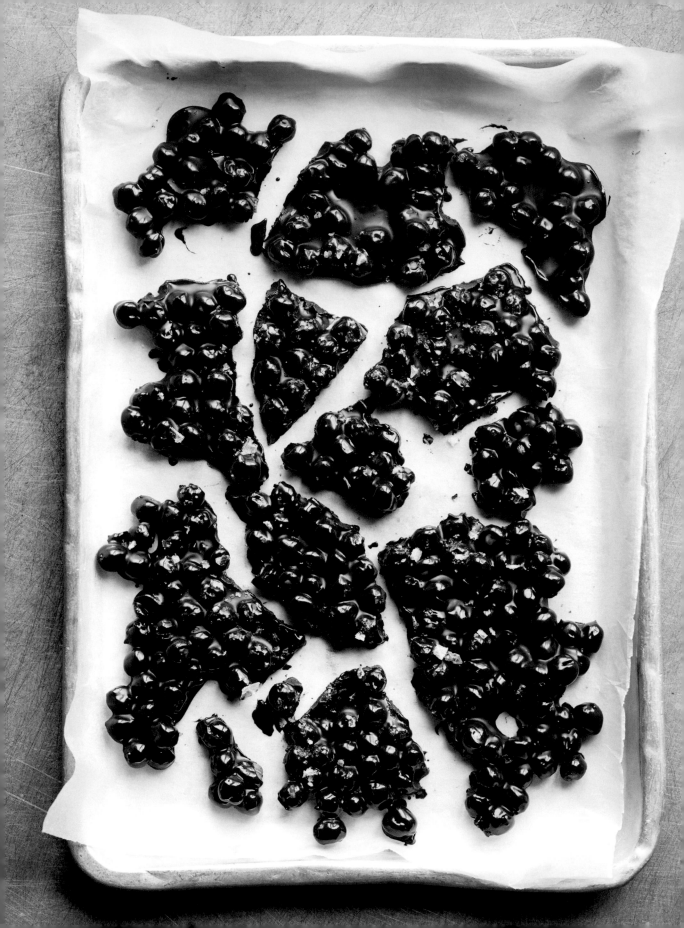

CHOCOLATE-COVERED ROASTED CHICKPEAS

PER SERVING | **168** CALS | **5G** PROTEIN | **7G** FAT | **20G** CARBS

5 MIN   30 MINS

SERVES 5

1 x 400g tin of
  chickpeas, drained
100g dark chocolate
  (at least 70% cacao)
a pinch of sea salt

An inexpensive and easy-to-make snack with only three ingredients, perfect for a mid-afternoon pick-me-up.

1 Preheat the oven to 200°C. Tip the drained chickpeas on to a baking tray, pat them dry with a tea towel or some kitchen roll and spread them out. Roast for 25–30 minutes until they're crispy and dry. Leave to cool.

2 Melt the chocolate (you can do this in short bursts in the microwave or in a heatproof bowl over a saucepan of boiling water).

3 In a large bowl, combine the roasted chickpeas with the melted chocolate and a pinch of sea salt. Spread out on a lined baking tray and place in the freezer for 30 minutes until set. Break up and divide between five food bags/containers. They will keep for up to 5 days in the fridge or up to 3 months in the freezer.

PROTEIN BALLS 3 WAYS

PER SERVING | **158** CALS | **6G** PROTEIN | **7G** FAT | **16G** CARBS

10 MINS · FREEZE

MAKES 10 PROTEIN BALLS

20g vanilla protein powder
30g coconut sugar
   or brown sugar
50g almonds
30g pecan nuts
100g large rolled oats
a pinch of salt
15g honey
75g pitted dates,
   roughly chopped
30g nut butter
   (I use almond)
1 tsp vanilla extract
semi-skimmed milk

The basic recipe here is for vanilla protein balls, and below are two other variations to tantalize those taste buds.

1 Put the protein powder, coconut or brown sugar, almonds and pecans into a food processor along with half the rolled oats and the salt. Blitz until you have a grainy mixture.

2 Add the honey, dates, nut butter and vanilla extract and blitz again, then tip the mixture into a bowl and stir in the remaining oats by hand.

3 Add 6–8 tablespoons of milk until you have a dough-like consistency. Roll the mixture into 10 balls. They will keep in the fridge for up to 3 days or in the freezer for up to 3 months.

VARIATION 1: CHOCOLATE ORANGE PROTEIN BALLS

Follow steps 1 and 2 above, then stir in the **zest and juice of half an orange** and **1 tablespoon of cocoa powder**. If the mixture is still a little dry, add 1–2 tablespoons of milk. Roll the mixture into 10 balls. They will keep in the fridge for up to 3 days or in the freezer for up to 3 months.

VARIATION 2: COCONUT PROTEIN BALLS

Follow steps 1 and 2 above, then stir in **15g of melted coconut oil**. If the mixture is still a little dry, add 1–2 tablespoons of milk. Roll the mixture into 10 balls, dampen with water and roll in **20g of desiccated coconut** until fully coated. They will keep in the fridge for up to 3 days or in the freezer for up to 3 months.

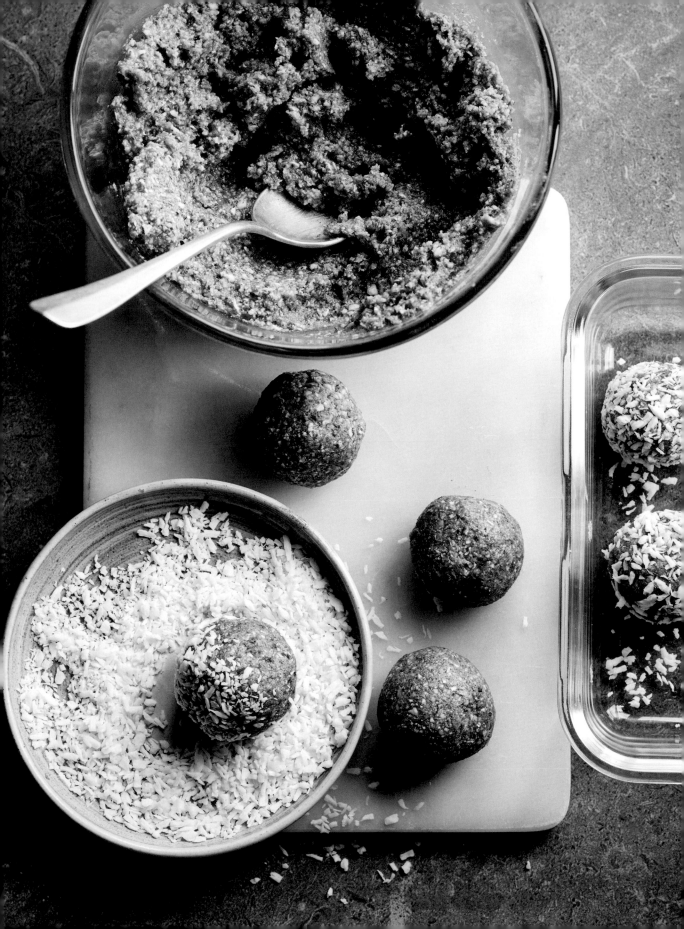

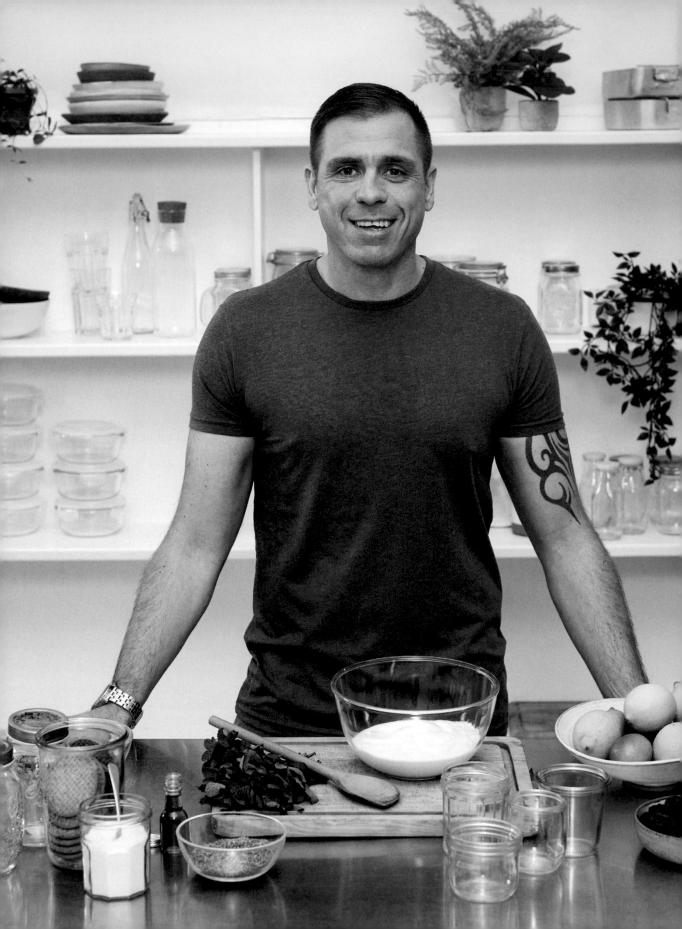

ACKNOWLEDGEMENTS

I'd like to express special thanks to the following people for their part in the realization of this endeavour.

First and foremost, Charlotte Deniz, for being a supporting and loving partner, for believing in me when no one else did and for being such an important and special part of this journey with me.

Frank Barrow for helping me fall in love with cooking and teaching me the fundamentals of cookery.

Stephen Orton for also believing in me when no one else did. He's a true friend who gave great advice and guidance throughout this whole journey.

It goes without saying, I would like to thank all the people at Michael Joseph and Penguin Random House on the teams that made this book happen, including anyone who worked on the book in the background that I haven't met.

I'd also like to thank Charlie Brotherstone, my book agent, who made all this possible; Grace Paul, who helped pull everything together; and the team who worked on the photo shoot and design, including Emma and Alex Smith, Jamie Orlando-Smith, Phil Mundy, Cynthia Blackett, Annie Swain and her assistants, and Malin Coleman. I hope I haven't forgotten anyone!

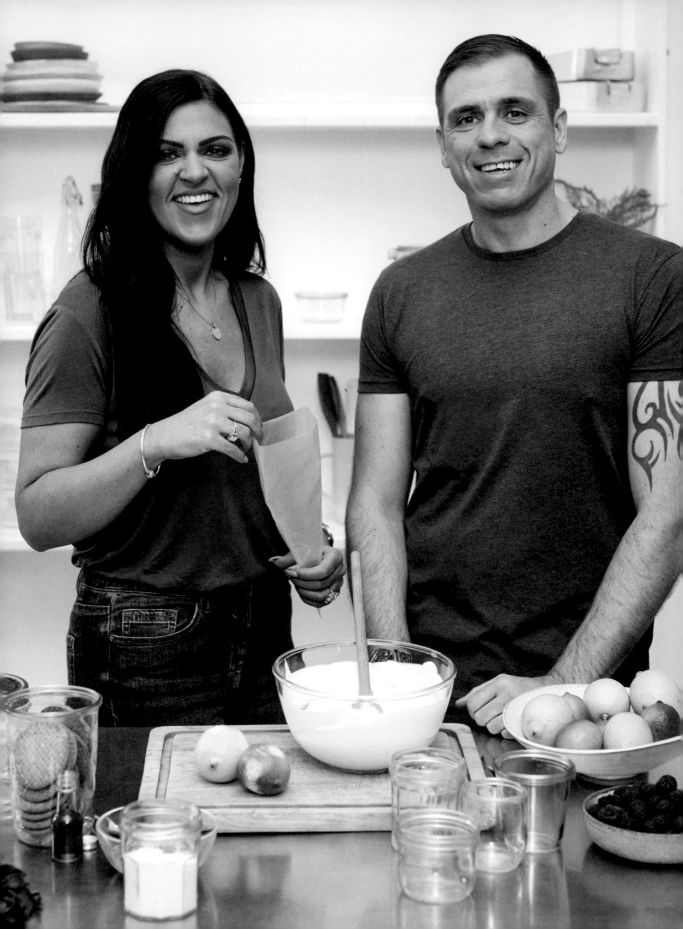

INDEX

MICHAEL JOSEPH

UK | USA | Canada | Ireland | Australia
India | New Zealand | South Africa

Michael Joseph is part of the Penguin Random House group of companies
whose addresses can be found at global.penguinrandomhouse.com

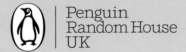

First published 2020
001

Copyright © The Meal Prep King Ltd, 2020
Photography copyright © Jamie Orlando Smith, 2020

The moral right of the author has been asserted

Set in Neutraface
Design and Art Direction by Smith & Gilmour Ltd
Photography by Jamie Orlando Smith
Food Stylist: Phil Mundy
Props Stylist: Cynthia Blackett
Colour reproduction by Altaimage Ltd
Printed and bound in China by C&C Offset Printing Co., Ltd

A CIP catalogue record for this book is available from the British Library

ISBN: 978-0-241-45312-4

www.greenpenguin.co.uk

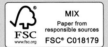

Penguin Random House is committed to a
sustainable future for our business, our readers
and our planet. This book is made from Forest
Stewardship Council® certified paper.

PRAISE FOR THE MEAL PREP KING

Thank you so much for sharing this. I'm a student nurse and I find it hard to plan healthy but tasty meals for 12-hour shifts. This will make a difference. **pamskella**

The recipes are easy to follow and taste amazing. It's the first time I've not dreaded what I'm going to have to eat on whatever daft diet I'm following. I've got about 5 stone to lose and I feel positive that I'm going to do it. **Samwilliams1990x**

I'm a mum of six and sometimes it's just so much easier to feed us a cheaper unhealthy diet. I am so glad I came across your page and am looking forward to following your tips and tricks!!! **Cluhhhrrissuhhh**

Meal prep this week has meant: less food waste, less time thinking about what to eat and less messing about clearing up and cooking each night. But mostly 3 lb down as I feel more in control and am not snacking or grabbing something quick, so THANK YOU! **Gwerdavies**

Thank you both for assisting in my love of cooking again. **Dawnbwrt**

I'm a midwife, so the meal prep is perfect for long shifts and means I'm not stopping on the way home for food as I know my dinner is waiting for me! **Ryoung135**

Taking the guesswork out of being healthy is priceless, especially to a super-busy mom like me! **chances_sj**

A gamechanger for my week! **Eimear.mccauley**

Normal food, no magic pills, teas, etc. – just proper food. **Angela Streeter**

This whole meal prepping thing makes our life so much easier in the long run. **Demi Labrea Plant**

PRAISE FOR THE MEAL PREP KING

Absolutely delicious! **Julia_cranny71**

Wow, definitely one of the best pages on IG. Great meal preps. **sine_g**

So inspiring! Thank you. Meal prep is key to attaining goals. **earth.to.laurie**

We've only been doing this for two days and it's been amazing. **Tracey Parsons**

I'm quite excited about planning next week's meals. Thank you for giving
me the inspiration to get off my bum and do something. **Janet Neill**

If all the meals are as delicious as this then I can't wait to fully
prep the weekend! **Lynn Gilding**

TMPK all the way, it's the future. Thanks, so much for the inspiration.
We can do this. **Lynda Lulu Ashworth**

Never found prepping and sticking to my calorie goals so easy
and tasty. **Samantha Neville**

Loving these recipes. Another six meals done. I'm making more than I'm consuming
each day to build up my prepped food. Thanks, TMPK! **Frank Osborne**

Thanks, guys, for restoring my love of cooking again. **s99urr**

I can't wait for my containers to come so I can get started.
Your food looks amazing! **Emma Meyrick**

Thank you for the recipes. Hubby loves them and this
will save us a fortune making our own! **Evie McCubbin**

I did my meal prep on Thursday and I'm loving it so far.
Wish I'd done this years ago! **Francine Burtenshaw**

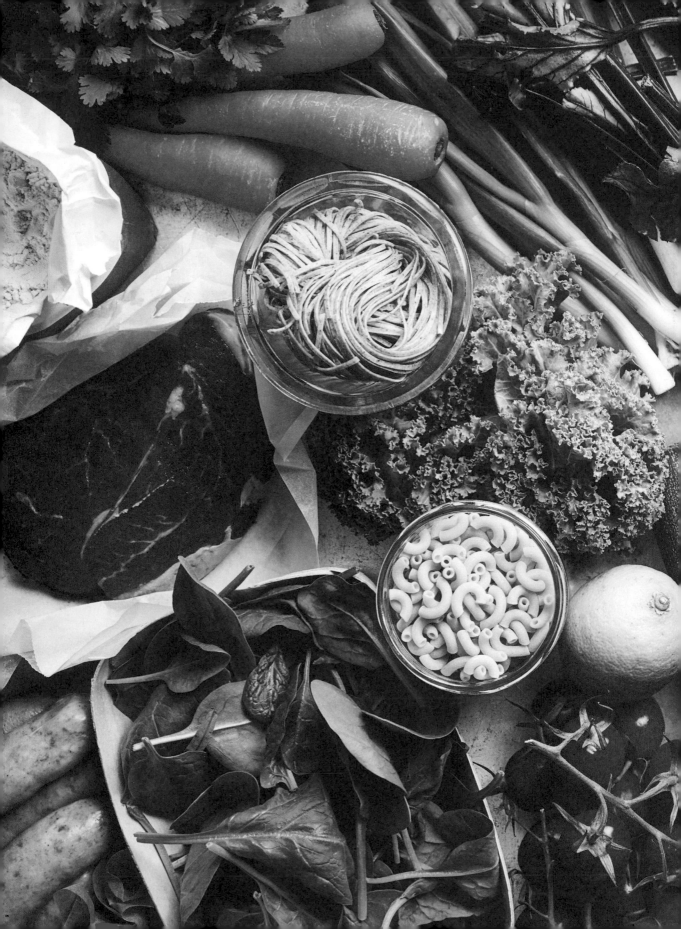